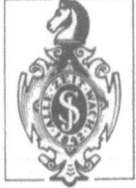

Treatment in Clinical Medicine
Series Editor: John L. Reid

David Parkes · Peter Jenner
David Rushton · David Marsden

Neurological Disorders

Springer-Verlag
London Berlin Heidelberg New York
Paris Tokyo

J. D. Parkes, MD, FRCP (Lond.)
Reader in Neurology, University Department of Neurology,
King's College School of Medicine and Dentistry, and Institute of
Psychiatry, London SE5 9RS

P. Jenner, BPharm, PhD, MPS
Reader in Neurochemical Pharmacology, University Department
of Neurology, Institute of Psychiatry, London SE5 8AF

D. N. Rushton, MD, MRCP
Honorary Consultant Neurologist, University Department of
Neurology, King's College School of Medicine and Dentistry, and
Institute of Psychiatry, London SE5 9RS

C. D. Marsden, DSc, FRCP, FRS
Professor of Neurology, University Department of Neurology,
King's College School of Medicine and Dentistry, and Institute of
Psychiatry, London SE5 9RS

ISBN-13: 978-3-540-17013-6   e-ISBN-13: 978-1-4471-3140-3
DOI: 10.1007/978-1-4471-3140-3

Library of Congress Cataloging-in-Publication Data
Neurological disorders.
(Treatment in clinical medicine) Includes bibliographies and index. 1. Nervous
system – Chemotherapy. I. Parkes, J.D. (J.David) II. Series. [DNLM: 1. Nervous
System Diseases – therapy. WL 100 N49455] RC349.8.N47   1987   616.8'0461
86–31652

Softcover reprint of the hardcover 1st edition 1987

The use of registered names, trademarks, etc. in this publication does not imply,
even in the absence of a specific statement, that such names are exempt from the
relevant protective laws and regulations and therefore free for general use.

Product Liability: The publisher can give no guarantee for information about drug
dosage and application thereof contained in this book. In every individual case the
respective user must check its accuracy by consulting other pharmaceutical
literature.

Typeset by Wilmaset, Birkenhead, Wirral
Printed by Page Bros (Norwich) Ltd, Mile Cross Lane, Norwich

2128/3916-543210

Series Editor's Foreword

Neurological Disorders is the latest and fifth monograph in the series on management and treatment in major clinical specialties or patient groups. Each book is complete in its own right and has been prepared by practising physicians with an interest in treatment and management, together with scientists involved in clinical research. The volumes are intended to fill a gap between standard textbooks of medicine and therapeutics and research reviews, symposia and original articles in superspecialist fields. It is the aim of the series to give authoritative up-to-date advice on treatment and management which will be of use to both specialists and nonspecialists and to allow recent advances in pathophysiology and developments in treatment to be viewed in the context of contemporary clinical practice. The approach is intentionally didactic. Each volume has been written by the minimum number of authors to ensure a degree of continuity and uniformity of style. The first four volumes dealt respectively with gastrointestinal diseases, rheumatic diseases, treatment in the elderly and cardiovascular disease. The present volume covers neurological diseases.

Chapter 1 is an introduction to drugs and the nervous system. It reviews the chemical basis of neurotransmission and mechanisms of drug action in neurological disease. There follows a series of chapters discussing patient management in general and drug treatment in particular in common neurological problems presenting in general medical practice. These include headache, cerebral vascular disease, epilepsy and the movement disorders. There is also a chapter on sleep and wakefulness which will be of general interest outwith the field of neurological disease. Other chapters cover infection in the nervous system and its drug management, and also the treatment of disease with immunosuppressants and cytotoxics. Management of disorders of peripheral nerves is covered in chapters on nerve and muscle diseases and a separate chapter on autonomic neuropathy. Finally, the role of drug treatment in neuroendocrinology is reviewed as is the role of vitamins and nutritional factors in neurological disease.

The authors work at the Department of Neurology at King's College Hospital and the Institute of Psychiatry in London where Dr. J.D. Parkes is Departmental Reader and Honorary Consultant Neurologist and Professor C.D. Marsden is Professor of Neurology. Dr. D.N. Rushton is a member of Scientific Staff, MRC Neurological Prostheses Unit and Honorary Consultant Neurologist, and Dr. P. Jenner is Reader in the Department of Neurology at the Institute of Psychiatry. The authors are thus well qualified to cover aspects of pathogenesis and underlying mechanisms, investigative management and drug treatment of patients with neurological disease. The book should provide a useful grounding in neurology for young doctors in training and studying for higher qualifications, and an update for a more experienced general physician or general practitioner who wishes to keep in touch with developments in neurology.

Glasgow, October 1986   John L. Reid

Preface

This book contains a dogmatic account of how we ourselves treat the neurological disorders we encounter every day. The contents reflect the frequency of hypertension and diabetes as well as headache and epilepsy in any neurological clinic; as well as our special interests in movement disorders, sleep and wakefulness, and the autonomic nervous system. Consideration of treatment of rare conditions, and critical discussion, have had to be omitted in a book of this nature.

Ideally, treatment in neurology should not be empirical, but founded on knowledge of the pharmacological properties of drugs. Throughout the book therefore we have emphasised points where this knowledge contributes to successful treatment. This book is intended primarily for junior hospital doctors and general practitioners. We think it will also be helpful to neurologists in training and to our medical colleagues.

Acknowledgement

We should like to thank all those who helped us with producing this book, and in particular to Lesley Gibson for all the time and effort she put into organising the chapters and typing the manuscript.

Contents

1 Drugs and the Nervous System

Neurones possess a variety of basic processes to ensure chemical neurotransmission. All of these processes provide targets for drug-induced manipulation of the nervous system. (a) Neurones synthesise and store one or more neurotransmitters. (b) Neurones release the neurotransmitter into the synaptic cleft in a pulsatile manner in response to impulse flow; but also limit its activity by reuptake into the neurone or by degradation. (c) Neurones regulate their own function through local feedback systems via events occurring in the synaptic cleft or via long loop feedback systems operating through neuronal contacts.

Neurotransmitters in the Nervous System

At a theoretical level the nervous system could function using two neurotransmitters—one causing excitation and the other inhibition. However, in practice the number of substances acting as neurotransmitters or neuromodulators within the nervous system is large. Six substances (acetylcholine, adrenaline, noradrenaline, dopamine, 5-hydroxytryptamine and GABA) are proven neurotransmitters. Pharmacological manipulation of these systems can be achieved and applied therapeutically. Many other substances are contained within clearly defined and localised neuronal networks yet the ability to alter their function is more limited than with the six classical neurotransmitters. The brain contains a variety of putative amino acid transmitters, particularly glutamate, aspartate and glycine. Only recently have selective synthetic agonists and antagonists of these substances become available.

Many neuropeptides have been demonstrated within the brain. Relatively little is understood of the mechanisms which control their synthesis or degradation and their role in brain function is unknown. Some neuropeptides are localised in the same neurone as classical neurotransmitters (e.g. cholecystokinin and dopamine; TRH and acetylcholine) but the relevance of this is not clear. However, the regional concentration of neuropeptides in brain is altered in a number of neurological and psychiatric diseases. The future development of synthetic neuropeptide agonist and antagonist drugs may provide a new range of treatments for neurological and psychiatric disorders.

A whole variety of other substances, including hormones, histamine, tryptamine, purines and prostaglandins, influence the function of the nervous system. Much research is being undertaken to find endogenous substrates for receptor sites in brain at which drugs act, but for which there is no known transmitter substance. A specific example is the search for an endogenous ligand for the benzodiazepine receptor; this may prove to be a β-carboline.

Neurotransmitter Receptors in the Nervous System

The ability of neurotransmitters to interact with receptor molecules which form part of the membrane of a neurone and to alter the electrical activity of that cell forms the basis of neurotransmission. Receptors are frequently considered as static "dents" in the surface of a membrane. They are in fact dynamic and complex macromolecules which can rapidly change in number or sensitivity. Also, the interaction between receptor and neurotransmitter is a dynamic process. The interaction results in a weak, not strong, bond which, as a necessary component of the pulsatile nature of neurotransmission can be rapidly reversed. Drugs acting at neurotransmitter receptors have a greater affinity for the receptor than the natural transmitter substance. A consequence of this increased affinity is that drug action is often prolonged or indeed in some circumstances is only terminated by the formation of new receptors.

Specific receptors are often considered to be located on the cell body of a neurone in the immediate proximity of the terminals of a contiguous neurone from which the specific neurotransmitter is released. In fact the receptors for a given neurotransmitter are located at presynaptic as well as postsynaptic sites. Presynaptic (or "auto") receptors are thought to be concerned with the self-regulation of neuronal function.

In addition to the neurotransmitter agonist or antagonist effect of drugs, there may be influences on neuronal activity by many other mechanisms:

1. The formation of cyclic nucleotides, such as cyclic AMP or cyclic GMP, via neurotransmitter stimulation of specific enzymes, such as adenylate cyclase or guanylate cyclase, may be necessary at some synapses to initiate the final impulse flow: here nucleotides can be influenced by drugs such as phosphodiesterase inhibitors (caffeine, aminophylline and rolipram) which prevent their breakdown.

2. Neurotransmission involves many enzyme-mediated reactions which require many different cofactors (e.g. tetrahydrobiopterin, heavy metals and active forms of niacin) and so are vulnerable to drug action.

3. The presence of ion channels or ionophores provides another site at which drug action occurs.

4. "Modulatory" sites are known to occur in close proximity to the primary neurotransmitter receptor. Drug action here may "tune" the response of the neurone to the neurotransmitter.

The GABA receptor complex is a good example of a receptor complex. Muscimol and bicuculline act at the recognition site; picrotoxin and some barbiturates at the ionophore site; and benzodiazepines at the modulatory site.

Factors Influencing Drug Action on the Nervous System

One important property of a drug which affects its ability to enter the brain and other parts of the nervous system is lipid solubility. The lipid-soluble form of a drug molecule is its nonionised state. The degree of drug ionisation is determined by pH. The ability of many drugs to penetrate into brain depends on their occurrence in a lipid-soluble nonionised form at physiological pH. The presence of the blood–brain barrier provides a natural means of limiting the actions of some drugs to the periphery (see e.g. cholinomimetic drugs and acetylcholine antagonists; Chap. 9).

Some drugs reach the brain by using active transport processes. This applies in particular to naturally occurring compounds, such as levodopa or L-tryptophan, or drugs which bear a strong structural resemblance to these compounds. Active transport may be limited by the amount of carrier available with saturation of the transport process or competition between alternative substrates, e.g. between levodopa and other amino acids. Drug action on the nervous system may be competitive (i.e. with an action that is readily reversible and can be overcome in the presence of another compound acting at the same site) or noncompetitive (with an effect that is not readily reversible nor is it surmounted by other drugs acting at the same site: this situation commonly exists with drugs blocking enzyme activity, e.g. monoamine oxidase inhibitors).

Drug Action on Neurotransmitter Mechanisms

Neurotransmitter Synthesis

Drug treatment can be used to enhance or inhibit the synthesis of transmitter substances. Where substrate availability for a synthetic enzyme is limited or the enzyme is not saturated by available substrate then administration of a transmitter precursor may enhance the concentration of the neuroactive substance. For example, administration of L-tryptophan can lead to an increase in brain 5-HT content since the enzyme tryptophan hydroxylase is not saturated by endogenous tryptophan. Similarly, the administration of L-dopa causes an increase in brain dopamine content because the enzyme concerned, namely L-aromatic amino acid decarboxylase, is present in large amounts. Administration of transmitter precursors does not always have the desired effect. Thus, administration of choline, deanol or lecithin may increase peripheral acetylcholine levels, but has little effect within the brain.

Inhibitors of transmitter synthesis exist for a variety of neuronal systems, but few of these compounds have any clinical use. α-Methyl-*para*-tyrosine inhibits the activity of tyrosine hydroxylase, the rate-limiting enzyme in the synthesis of dopamine, and has been employed in the treatment of catecholamine-producing tumours. Noradrenaline synthesis can be inhibited by dopamine β-hydroxylase inhibitors (e.g. disulfiram) and 5-HT synthesis by the tryptophan hydroxylase inhibitor, *para*-chlorophenylalanine. A further use of enzyme inhibitors is illustrated by the ability of selective inhibitors of peripheral L-aromatic amino acid decarboxylase (e.g. carbidopa or benserazide) to prevent the breakdown of orally administered L-dopa, so allowing its passage into brain.

Neurotransmitter Storage

A number of drugs disrupt neuronal storage mechanisms for the monoamine transmitters adrenaline, noradrenaline, dopamine and 5-HT. Reserpine acts by causing a disruption of long-term granular stores of all monoamines. This effect is of long duration since the storage granules have to be resynthesised. Compounds such as tetrabenazine and oxypertine also disrupt monoamine storage, but affect dopamine, noradrenaline and 5-HT differentially. The effects of tetrabenazine and oxypertine are short-lasting and reversible. It is likely these drugs act on mobile rather than long-term transmitter stores.

Neurotransmitter Release

The release of a neurotransmitter in response to an action potential usually occurs by the process of exocytosis initiated by the entry of calcium ions into the neuronal terminals. Drugs can influence the process of transmitter release in a number of ways:

1. Compounds such as ephedrine, phenylpropanolamine, α-methyldopa and amphetamine can increase the release of monoamine transmitters from storage sites. (These drugs may also act as "false" transmitters which displace the endogenous transmitter molecules.)

2. Inhibition of noradrenaline release can be produced by drugs such as guanethidine and bretylium. The mechanism involved is not clear.

3. Stabilisation of the neuronal membrane or interference with calcium ion transport may prevent transmitter release (e.g. nifedipine and verapamil).

Neurotransmitter Reuptake

The action of neurotransmitters released into the synaptic cleft is terminated by (a) reuptake into the neurone and (b) enzymatic degradation. Most neuronal systems possess selective high-affinity, sodium-dependent uptake systems for their transmitter substance; these can be inhibited by drug treatment.

At present only the reuptake of the monoamines dopamine, noradrenaline and 5-HT is known to be affected by drugs in current clinical use. The best known of these are the tricyclic antidepressants, (e.g. imipramine, desipramine and amitriptyline). These compounds are relatively nonselective in their effects on the different monoamines. However, recently highly selective drugs altering either noradrenaline uptake (e.g. maprotiline) or 5-HT uptake (e.g. fluoxetine and zimelidine) have been introduced.

Neurotransmitter Degradation

Specific examples of enzyme systems involved in transmitter breakdown include acetylcholine esterase (breakdown of acetylcholine to choline) and monoamine oxidase and catecholamine o-methyl transferase (breakdown of dopamine to homovanillic acid and 3,4-dihydroxyphenylacetic acid). The breakdown of the monoamine transmitters, adrenaline, noradrenaline, dopamine and 5-HT, is reversibly or irreversibly prevented by monoamine oxidase inhibitors. The enzyme exists as two isoenzymes, monamine oxidase A and B, with a different substrate selectivity. (In the human brain, monoamine oxidase A: noradrenaline and 5-HT; monoamine oxidase B: dopamine). Some monoamine oxidase inhibitors act on both enzymes in the dosages in clinical use (e.g. pargyline, tranylcypromine and nialamide). However, eldepryl in low doses (e.g. below 50 mg daily) selectively inhibits monoamine oxidase B, and clorgyline monoamine oxidase A.

The breakdown of acetylcholine is prevented by inhibitors of acetylcholine esterase, such as physostigmine, neostigmine and succinylcholine. Recently, inhibitors of the GABA-metabolising enzyme GABA transaminase, namely γ-acetylenic GABA and γ-vinyl GABA, have been examined for the possible treatment of epilepsy.

Neurotransmitter Receptors

Neurotransmitter agonists (drugs which mimic the action of another compound) and antagonists which act on the classical monoamine systems, cholinergic, GABAergic, excitatory amino acid and opiate systems are known. Few synthetic compounds acting on other peptide systems have been described.

The classification of agonist (and antagonist) compounds is as follows:

1. Complete agonist—having the same effect as the natural neurotransmitter

2. Partial agonist—producing a submaximal effect or with dose dependency producing mixed agonist–antagonist actions

3. Inverse agonist—some compounds acting on benzodiazepine receptors in the manner expected of an agonist, producing antagonist functional effects

Examples of neurotransmitter agonist and antagonist drugs for the major neurotransmitter systems are given in Table 1.1. Multiple forms of many neurotransmitter receptors are believed to exist. Examples of the classification of neurotransmitter receptors are given in Table 1.2. For some neurotransmitter subtypes selective drugs are in current clinical use and examples are given in Table 1.3.

Table 1.1. Agonist and antagonist drugs for neurotransmitter receptors

Receptor type	Agonist	Antagonist
Adrenergic	Phenylephrine Isoprenaline Clonidine Salbutamol	Phentolamine Phenoxybenzamine Prazosin Propranolol
Dopaminergic	Apomorphine Bromocriptine Pergolide Lisuride	Chlorpromazine Haloperidol Flupenthixol Sulpiride
5-HT	Ritanserin LSD Other hallucinogens	Methergoline Cyproheptadine Mianserin
Histaminergic	Betazole	Mepyramine Diphenhydramine Cimetidine Ranitidine
Cholinergic	Carbachol Pilocarpine	Atropine Scopolamine Mecamylamine
GABA	Muscimol	Bicuculline Picrotoxin
Opiate	Morphine Pentazocine Ethylketocyclazocine	Naloxone Naltrexone Nalorphine

Table 1.2. Classification of multiple forms of neurotransmitter receptors

Receptor system	Receptor subtypes
Adrenergic	α_1, α_2 β_1, β_2
Dopaminergic	D-1_L, D-1_H D-2_L, D-2_H
5-HT	5-HT$_{1A}$, 5-HT$_{1B}$ 5-HT$_2$
Histaminergic	H-1, H-2
Cholinergic	Muscarinic (M-1, M-2) Nicotinic
GABA	GABA$_A$, GABA$_B$ (also ionophore and benzodiazepine sites)
Opiate	Sigma, mu, delta, kappa

Table 1.3. Examples of compounds selective for receptor subtypes

Receptor subtype	Agonist	Antagonist
Adrenergic		
α-1	Oxymetazoline	Prazosin
α-2		Yohimbine
β-1	Isoprenaline	Atenolol
β-2		Butoxamine
Dopaminergic		
D-1	SKF 38393	SCH 23390
D-2	Bromocriptine	Sulpiride
5-HT		
5-HT$_{1A}$	8-Hydroxy-DPAT	(−)-Pindolol
5-HT$_{1B}$	RU 24969	
5-HT$_2$	Hallucinogens	Ritanserin
Histaminergic		
H-1		Mepyramine
H-2		Cimetidine
Cholinergic		
Muscarinic M-1		Pirenzepine
Muscarinic M-2		
Nicotinic	Cytisine	Mecamylamine
GABA		
GABA$_A$	Muscimol	Bicuculline
GABA$_B$	Baclofen	
Opiate		
Delta	DADLE	ICI 154,129
Kappa	Ethylketocyclazocine	Quadrazocine
Mu	Fentanyl	Naloxone
Sigma	Benzmorphans	

Adaptation of the Nervous System to Drug Treatment

The repeated administration of a drug can lead to alterations in the response elicited. Such change can be induced by alterations in the pharmacokinetic handling of drugs owing to processes such as enzyme induction or inhibition. But the nervous system itself can respond in a number of ways to chronic drug treatment so as to alter the nature of the pharmacological response obtained.

Chronic drug treatment may cause central nervous system adaptation in two ways:

1. Alterations in presynaptic events
2. Alterations in the response of neurotransmitter receptors

Examples are as follows:

1. Following treatment with reserpine, the activity of tyrosine hydroxylase is increased so as to overcome the loss of transmitter incurred. In contrast, the administration of neuroleptic drugs, which act acutely by blocking brain dopamine receptors, causes a compensatory presynaptic increase in dopamine synthesis and release in an attempt to overcome the inhibition of dopamine receptor function. On repeated administration the initial increase in tyrosine hydroxylase activity shows tolerance, such that dopamine synthesis returns to normal.

2. Classical pharmacology of the neuromuscular junction dictates that a reduction in neurotransmission causes an increase in receptor numbers causing receptor supersensitivity, whereas repeated application of the neurotransmitter or an agonist will cause a decrease or "down-regulation" of receptor numbers.

Many antidepressant drugs act by blockade of noradrenaline reuptake on acute administration so increasing transmitter concentrations in the synaptic cleft. However, on repeated administration the effect of enhanced bombardment of postsynaptic receptors by noradrenaline is to lead to a down-regulation of the β-receptor. This effect takes days or weeks to occur as does the onset of antidepressant activity.

Neuroleptic drugs block brain dopamine receptors on acute drug administration. However, on chronic drug administration dopamine receptor blockade disappears and dopamine receptor supersensitivity appears. This mechanism is a response of the receptor to the loss of transmitter action. With neuroleptic drugs, the initial compensatory change may be functionally related to antipsychotic activity, with the subsequent development of tardive dyskinesia as a result of dopamine receptor overactivity.

Further Reading

Batchelard HS (1981) Brain biochemistry. Chapman and Hall, London

Cooper JR, Bloom FE, Roth RH (1982) The biochemical basis of neuropharmacology, 4th edn. Oxford University Press, New York

Gilman A, Goodman LS, Rall TW, Murad F (eds) (1985) Goodman and Gilman's the pharmacological basis of therapeutics, 7th edn. MacMillan, New York

Iversen SD, Iversen LL (1981) Behavioural pharmacology, 2nd edn. Oxford University Press, Oxford

Kruk ZL, Pycock CJ (1983) Neurotransmitters and drugs, 2nd edn. Croom Helm, London

Tyrer PJ (ed) (1982) Drugs in psychiatric practice. Butterworths, London.

2 Headache, Pain and Raised Intracranial Pressure

Common migraine, tension-vascular headache, tension headache and "ordinary" headache overlap, and clinical diagnosis is not exact. Classic migraine and REM sleep-locked cluster headache are distinct clinical entities that can be easily recognised.

Tension Headache

Stress, fatigue, visual glare or noise are common causes of headache. This is often attributed to muscle tension or vasodilatation, and a vicious circle of muscle tension and pain is often postulated. When pain and muscle tension in neck or scalp are found to coexist, therefore, it is hard to determine which was the original cause of the vicious circle. However, scalp-muscle EMG activity is often entirely normal in patients considered to have "tension" headache.

If tension factors cannot be avoided, and treatment of psychological factors is not effective then simple analgesics, such as aspirin or other single-ingredient preparations should be used (Table 2.1). Headache is a common cause of analgesic abuse, and chronic treatment with aspirin or paracetamol may lead to nephritis or peptic ulceration. Minor tranquillisers (e.g. chlordiazepoxide (5–30 mg/day), diazepam (2–30 mg/day), or flunitrazepam 0.125 mg nightly) occasionally relieve stress headache. Tricyclic antidepressant drugs (e.g. dothiepin 50–150 mg at night, amitriptyline 25–150 mg at night) may give dramatic relief from chronic tension headache in depressed patients, but are also sometimes very effective in patients who are not overtly depressed. Major tranquillisers and narcotic analgesics should be avoided. Reassurance and sometimes a normal CT scan with a simple explanation of the cause of the headache is often far more effective than prescription of yet another analgesic.

Table 2.1. Pain relief in neurology

Drug (mean oral dose)	Main uses	Major therapeutic problems
Aspirin 300–900 mg 4-hourly	Headache; superficial or bone pain; musculo-skeletal pain	Salicylism; gastric erosion; dyspepsia; hypersensitiv-ity reactions
Propionic acid derivatives, e.g. naproxen	As aspirin, but twice daily; lower incidence of toxic side effects	As aspirin
Flufenamic acid 200 mg 4-hourly Mefenamic acid derivatives	Moderate pain relief; little anti-inflammatory effect	Diarrhoea; haemolytic anaemia
Indomethacin 25–50 mg 2–3 times daily	Anti-inflammatory as well as analgesic; effective relief of migraine; night joint pain and night stiff-ness	Sometimes causes headache; gastrointesti-nal bleeding; haemato-logical problems; agranulocytosis
Phenylbutazone 200 mg 2–3 times daily (availability limited owing to toxicity)	Good pain relief in anky-losing spondylitis	Gastric bleeding; agranulo-cytosis; rarely fluid retention; cardiac failure
Codeine phosphate 30–60 mg 4-hourly	Pain in head injury; sub-arachnoid haemorrhage, etc.	Severe constipation
Morphine sulphate 10–20 mg	Severe pain; causes euphoria and mental detachment	Nausea; vomiting; respira-tory depression; consti-pation; hypertension
Diamorphine 5–10 mg	More potent than mor-phine	Very addictive; rapid toler-ance
Pethidine 50–100 mg	Short duration of action; probably drug of choice for relief of pain with intracranial damage, since little respiratory depression	As morphine; weaker analgesic
Buprenorphine 300–600 μg i.m. or slowly i.v. 3–4 times daily	Long duration of action; low dependence poten-tial	Not reversed by naloxone

Migraine

The following patterns are recognised:

1. Premonitory migraine, characterised by a feeling of good health, energy, thirst, hunger and sometimes drowsiness. This phase is often recognised only in retrospect.

2. Classic migraine, with a visual or other aura preceding unilateral headache by 10–60 min. The initial aura is attributed to vasoconstriction

which is sometimes limited to branches of one ophthalmic artery. Focal symptoms may persist into the headache phase, particularly in vertebrobasilar migraine (which is most common in females), as well as in childhood migraine and hemiplegic attacks.

3. Migraine prodromata may occur with no subsequent headache.

4. Nonprodromal migraine, usually with episodic, severe, protracted headache, often unilateral, prominent nausea and vomiting, and sometimes photophobia. Many cases of menstrual migraine are of this nature.

5. Tension headaches are common in patients with migraine.

The prodromata of migraine are usually accompanied by a reduction in regional cerebral blood flow, and the headache phase by increased cerebral and extracranial blood flow. Attacks may be associated with, or followed by, changes in plasma and platelet serotonin levels; serotonin causes vasoconstriction in some, but not all, cerebral blood vessels. Tyramine, a vasoactive amine present in many foods, dairy produce and fish, may trigger migraine in 10%– 30% of patients, but only in a small minority of patients does stopping these or other foods (such as chocolate, cheese or oranges) prevent attacks.

Migraine Prophylaxis

Biofeedback, relaxation training and other forms of psychological encouragement are usually unsuccessful, whilst drugs are simpler to prescribe, less time-consuming and more effective. Rebreathing into a paper bag can raise pCO_2 and hence cause cerebral vasodilatation. This can abort a migraine attack if used in the premonitory vasoconstrictor phase.

Migraine prophylaxis with drugs (Table 2.2) is used where headaches occur frequently (2–3 per month or more), and can be used in conjunction with treatment of any acute attacks that may occur in spite of prophylaxis. When attacks of migraine are less frequent, continuous prophylaxis is not usually worthwhile. Where migraines occur in well-defined bouts separated by migraine-free intervals, prophylaxis during the bouts only may be worthwhile. If prophylaxis is highly effective, then a trial withdrawal may be the only practical way to determine whether the bout has finished.

Apart from hormone-related (menstrual) migraine, it is not possible to predict which migraine prophylactic will be best, and it may be necessary to try several in sequence, each for an adequate length of time (1–3 months, depending on the frequency of attacks). Overall, migraine prophylaxis will reduce attack frequency and severity in two-thirds of all patients.

Ergot derivatives in low or high dosages are perhaps best avoided for migraine prophylaxis. Several other classes of drugs have been found to be effective prophylactics, although none is always effective.

Table 2.2. Prophylaxis and treatment of migraine

Drug (daily dose)	Indications	Adverse reactions	Contraindications
Propranolol 40–160 mg	Migraine; cluster headache	Heart failure, bronchoconstriction, depression, drowsiness	Heart failure, asthma
Cyproheptadine 4–16 mg	As propranolol	Drowsiness, anticholinergic effects	Glaucoma, prostatism
Tricyclic antidepressants (e.g. imipramine 25–150 mg)	Migraine associated with depression	Dry mouth, postural hypotension, cardiac arrhythmias	Coronary artery disease
Phenytoin 5 mg/kg	Possibly of benefit in some children with migraine	Drowsiness, ataxia, gingivitis, etc.	Effect not definitely established
Domperidone 10–20 mg	Menstrual migraine; prophylaxis and treatment of nausea and vomiting	Extremely rare acute dystonia	
Indomethacin 25–50 mg	Acute migraine headache	Gastrointestinal discomfort, headache, ulceration and bleeding, rarely drowsiness	Peptic ulcer, salicylate hypersensitivity; beware blood dyscrasias, particularly thrombocytopenia
Ergot derivatives	Acute attack only; use in limited dosage	Nausea, vasoconstriction, abortifacient; may perpetuate headache; ergotism	Vascular disease, pregnancy, hypertension, renal and hepatic disease

Beta-blockers (e.g. propranolol 30–120 mg daily in divided doses) will reduce anxiety as well as reducing peripheral vasospasm, and will reduce attack frequency in over 50% of patients. Antihistamines such as cyproheptadine 4–12 mg daily; or prochlorperazine 15–30 mg daily (beware extrapyramidal side effects) may help. Antidepressants, either tricyclic (e.g. amitriptyline 75 mg daily), or MAO inhibitors (e.g. phenelzine 15 mg three or four times daily: beware food–drug interactions) may be effective. Benzodiazepines (e.g. diazepam 2–30 mg daily) or indomethacin (25–50 mg daily) may be useful.

Menstrual migraine sometimes responds to diuretics (acetazolamide 250–500 mg daily in the premenstrual week) or depot oestrogens (oestradiol 25–50 mg implant). Oral contraceptives may either increase or decrease the frequency of migraine attacks.

The α-adrenergic agonist drug clonidine given in low dosage (tablets each containing 25 μg; 2–6 daily) is ineffective in our experience. Pizotifen 1.5 mg daily (a serotonin- and histamine-blocking drug) causes long-term improvement without serious side effects, although weight gain is an occasional problem.

The potent serotonin antagonist methysergide (2–6 mg daily) is an effective migraine prophylactic, and has been widely used for resistant cases in the past. It is now considered outdated and has been largely discarded, because it causes frequent and serious toxic effects similar to those of other ergot alkaloids, including the sinister condition of retroperitoneal fibrosis.

Treatment of the Acute Migraine Attack

Ergot derivatives (e.g. ergotamine 1 mg at the onset of attack, repeated once after 2 h if necessary) are the traditional treatment for the acute migraine attack. They are prescribed less freely than previously, with increasing awareness of the hazards of overdosage, particularly when, as is often the case, they are taken in ways and doses not intended by the prescribing physician.

Ergot derivatives are potent vasoconstrictors resulting occasionally in arterial damage, and are contraindicated in patients with ischaemic heart disease or peripheral vascular disease, as well as in pregnancy. Both overdosage with ergot derivatives and withdrawal of ergot derivatives given long-term can result in severe headache, which can easily be misinterpreted as a recurrence of migraine. Some cases of complicated migraine with persistent retinal or neurological deficit after the acute attack may result from ergot toxicity rather than from the vasoconstriction of migraine. Ergot derivatives for the acute attack should therefore be given only where attacks are severe, not relieved by other forms of treatment, and not too frequent (twice a week at most). It should be carefully emphasised that overdosage is dangerous, that not more than 3 mg ergotamine should be taken in any day or 6 mg in any week, and that it has been shown that in most people 1 mg ergotamine is as effective as any larger dose. Dihydroergotamine causes less nausea and vomiting than ergotamine and has less oxytocic effects, but loses potency rapidly in solution.

Nausea or sickness may be prevented by domperidone, 10–20 mg p.o. or i.m. Metoclopramide, 10–20 mg, is equally effective, but causes acute dystonic reactions in 2%–5% of the population. Indomethacin, 25–50 mg, or the anti-inflammatory drug flufenamic acid 200 mg, as well as other nonsteroidal anti-inflammatory drugs can be as effective as, and may be less toxic than, ergot derivatives. Analgesics may be combined with domperidone.

Migraine headache can sometimes be relieved by an ice bag on the head (which may induce reflex vasoconstriction) or by the no longer fashionable leech on the head (acting as a counterirritant). Bed rest in a dark quiet room is often necessary. Feverfew (2–4 small leaves or 1–2 large leaves every day) is a popular herbal remedy. The yellow-green leaves of this bushy plant, *Tanacetum parthenium*, are eaten either untreated or between two slices of bread and butter, usually mixed with honey to mask the strong and bitter flavour. Feverfew has been used even more for arthritis than migraine since the sixteenth century.

Migrainous Neuralgia

A not uncommon condition occurring mainly in males, migrainous neuralgia causes bouts of severe unilateral retro-orbital facial pain and headache lasting 1–2 h, often waking the patient from REM sleep, and thus most common in the last third of the night, when this sleep phase is most prevalent. There is profuse lachrymation and nose blockage. In the variant known as chronic paroxysmal hemicrania, attacks are more frequent, of shorter duration, and less clearly REM sleep-locked. Internal carotid, supraorbital and frontal artery blood flow is reduced during an episode of cluster pain. Attacks may be provoked by alcohol, nitroglycerine and occasionally by neck flexion or rotation.

Attacks can be prevented by indomethacin 25–75 mg daily; or prednisone 40 mg daily for 5 days and then reducing to 2–10 mg daily; or lithium carbonate 250 mg three times daily initial dose and then as determined by plasma levels; or dihydroergotamine, although tolerance to ergot derivatives sometimes develops.

Temporal Arteritis

Temporal (giant cell) arteritis is four times commoner in women than men, and occurs mainly, but not always in patients over the age of 55. It is associated with polymyalgia rheumatica in 30% of cases. Malaise, fever, anorexia and weight loss are common. The diagnosis is made in the presence of headache, with tenderness and oedema of the temples or occiput, usually but not always with a high ESR (over 40 mm/h). Arterial biopsy shows destruction of the arterial wall, and multinucleate giant cells, but patchy involvement ("skip lesions") may account for false-negative biopsies. If possible, a tender segment should be marked with a skin pencil before surgery. Involvement of extracranial rather than intracranial vessels is the rule, although the vertebral artery may be affected in the neck, and mesenteric and other vessels are sometimes affected. Steroid treatment is mandatory, since without it 20%–30% of patients go blind, usually owing to ciliary rather than retinal involvement. Other complications such as a third or sixth nerve palsy are less common. Pain often responds within 24 h of starting prednisolone 60–80 mg daily (preferably enteric-coated in 3–4 divided doses), but the ESR may not normalise for some weeks. Dosage may be reduced to 20 mg daily after 3 weeks, and thereafter is determined by the presence or absence of headache, and the elevation of the ESR. It is sometimes possible to tail off treatment after several months, but often it is necessary to continue for many months, years or for the lifetime. All hazards of chronic steroid treatment may occur, the most troublesome being a change in appearance, with considerable weight gain, and the most frightening, silent gastrointestinal perforation. The likelihood of complications can be minimised by maintenance on the smallest possible dose that keeps the patient symptom-free, with an alternate-day schedule.

Postherpetic Neuralgia

Herpes zoster (shingles) is caused by reactivation of latent varicella virus (chickenpox). This has a predilection for dorsal root and cranial ganglia, most often the gasserian and geniculate. Permanent burning, aching pain develops after shingles in up to 50% of elderly people. This may be prevented by treating the acute attack with analgesics such as aspirin, paracetamol or codeine. Steroids should be avoided. Treatment of the acute eruption with topical or systemic acyclovir (see p. 121) may radically shorten the duration of the attack, and limit painful sequelae.

Once postherpetic neuralgia is established, treatment is very difficult and requires considerable patience and persistence. Analgesics, sedatives and antidepressants (for example, carbamazepine 200–600 mg daily, and imipramine 25–100 mg daily) are all of occasional value. Physical treatment such as spraying the skin with ethyl chloride, subcutaneous or deeper injection of local anaesthetic, vibration and even deep X-ray therapy, may be worthwhile. Narcotic analgesics should be avoided. The antiviral drug amantadine is not of value. Polyethylene or Plastazote jackets can be obtained for patients whose pain is made worse by contact with clothing. Transcutaneous electrical stimulation (e.g. Devices Stimtech stimulator) used intelligently over long periods may replace the pain of postherpetic neuralgia by a more tolerable sensation, and very occasionally permanent pain relief is obtained. There is no place for nerve root division or other major surgical procedures.

Trigeminal Neuralgia

Trigeminal neuralgia is more common in old than young people, and in women then men. Pain involves the maxillary and mandibular divisions more commonly than the ophthalmic division of the trigeminal nerve, and is precipitated by touching or moving the face with specific trigger areas. Some 4% of cases are bilateral, and a few are due to brain stem or cerebellopontine angle disease. There is increasing evidence that most so-called idiopathic cases are due to sensory root compression, irritation and demyelination by blood vessels, often a hardened superior cerebellar artery.

Oral carbamazepine 300–1200 mg daily in three divided doses, phenytoin 200–400 mg, clonazepam 2–6 mg, and baclofen 10–80 mg daily, may be tried in that order. Usually, high doses are needed, relief is partial rather than complete, and side effects are not infrequent. Eventual escape from drug control requires surgery. The action of these drugs may be related to their ability to modify abnormal impulse generation and transmission in the gasserian ganglion and trigeminal sensory root, or to cause sedation. Glossopharyngeal neuralgia responds to these drugs as well as trigeminal neuralgia, but other forms of facial neuralgia do not. Pain relief rather than side effects should be used to determine dosage, since the side effects are reversible and dose-related, while the pain may lead to suicide. Carbamazepine should not be given to patients with atrioventricular conduction defects unless paced. It can occasionally give rise to jaundice and blood dyscrasias. However, these rare serious side effects occur only in patients who develop a skin rash when carbamazepine is started (about 3%). For this reason, the drug should always be withdrawn if a drug rash occurs. Because of the warning value of the drug rash, many physicians do not do routine liver function tests and blood counts on patients on carbamazepine.

If pain continues despite medical treatment, surgical denervation by nerve or ganglion injection, thermocoagulation of the gasserian ganglion, sensory root division or nerve decompression is required. For a young, fit patient, or in the presence of severe bilateral pain, the latter alternative is to be preferred. Thermocoagulation is however a safer and simpler procedure than posterior fossa craniotomy, and is very effective in relieving tic douloureux in 95% of patients. The pain often recurs after 3–5 years, and 2%–3% of patients develop anaesthesia dolorosa, sometimes as troublesome as the original pain. Distal nerve blocks are often unsatisfactory, with frequent pain recurrence or troublesome dysaesthesiae.

Other Facial Pains

Pain due to disease of the eyes, sinuses, teeth, or temporomandibular joint usually presents little diagnostic difficulty, although there is a bewildering group of patients with episodic or persistent unilateral or bilateral lower facial pain, who have no evidence of bad teeth or sinus infection, and no motor or sensory abnormalities to explain their symptoms. Antidepressant drug treatment of atypical facial pain is more often recommended than successful. Carotidynia is not a disease entity, but describes tenderness and pain in migraine, temporal arteritis, other vascular disorders, or following carotid surgery. A vascular mechanism has also been proposed for headache following excess stimulation of the trigeminal nerve (e.g. diving into cold water) or the glossopharyngeal nerve (ice cream headache).

Cervical Spondylosis Headache

Most diseases of the upper neck, which commonly cause pain, do so in cervical and occipital distribution, rather than causing vertex or frontal headache. The headache of cervical spondylosis may be due to both referred joint pain and muscle tension. It is improved by warmth, immobilisation, local anaesthetic injection into tender areas, indomethacin 25–75 mg daily, diazepam 5–30 mg daily, or soluble aspirin 300–900 mg 4-hourly. The neck–tongue syndrome (pain in the neck and ipsilateral tongue on sudden neck movement) is explained by irritation of the second cervical dorsal root, which carries common sensory fibres from the tongue via interconnections with the hypoglossal nerve. Irritation of the third cervical nerve is a common cause of occipital headache in cervical spondylosis.

Headache Due to Cerebral Oedema and Increased Intracranial Pressure

Headache, vomiting, papilloedema and focal neurological signs with tumour-related brain oedema respond to dexamethasone 20 mg daily in four divided doses; occasionally, higher doses up to 60 mg daily are given. Dexamethasone causes little salt retention. Overall, 80% of subjects with primary or secondary brain tumours are improved, but the favourable response usually lasts only a few weeks, and the ultimate prognosis is not altered. If a very rapid reduction of intracranial pressure is needed before surgery, the osmotic agents mannitol, glycerol, urea, or glucose 50% in water will quickly reduce brain water. Mannitol 1 g/kg given over 15 min reduces intracranial pressure by about 40% for 2–4 h, and causes a large osmotic diuresis (and hence a need for catheterisation). A subsequent rebound in intracranial pressure is usual.

Osmotic Treatment of Raised Intracranial Pressure

Urea, mannitol and glycerol are osmotic diuretics. They can, however, reduce raised intracranial pressure by a different mechanism, altering the osmotic gradient across the blood–brain barrier.

Urea

Urea, in sufficient concentrations (i.v. infusion 40–80 g as a 30% solution in glucose intravenous infusion 5%–10%, at a rate not exceeding 3–4 ml/min) will reduce the pressure and volume of the CSF, and reduce cerebral oedema, with transfer of water from the brain to the plasma. However, urea may slowly penetrate the brain, and a rebound rise in CSF pressure may occur after 4–6 h.

Mannitol and Glycerol

Mannitol and glycerol produce less rebound increase in intracranial pressure than urea, as they penetrate the brain more slowly. Mannitol has a more potent and rapid action than glycerol. Glycerol is used mainly before ophthalmic surgery, to lower intraocular pressure. It is rapidly metabolised, being a substrate for glycolysis. It has a gluconeogenic and antiketotic effect, so it can cause nonketotic hyperglycaemia and even coma if given long-term to diabetic subjects. Mannitol must be given i.v. A rapid infusion of 1.5–2 g/kg over 30–60 min before surgery will shrink the brain when this is required by the surgeon. The CSF pressure falls within 15 min of starting injection, with maximum reduction at 30–60 min. For a more prolonged action, 50–200 g infused in 24 h will reduce elevated intracranial and intraocular pressure. Mannitol is not metabolised, but is cleared by glomerular filtration, with little tubular reabsorption. Toxicity is due to disturbance of water and electrolyte balance; Na^+, K^+ and water are lost in the osmotic diuresis. It should not be given to patients with intracerebral haemorrhage unless surgery is going to be performed, and infusion should be stopped if the patient develops signs of heart failure, pulmonary congestion or progressive renal dysfunction. If mannitol accumulates in renal failure, it will expand the extracellular fluid volume and cause water intoxication, with congestive cardiac failure, pulmonary oedema, oedema, hypertension, electrolyte depletion, acidosis, dry mouth, thirst, blurred vision, thrombophlebitis, convulsions, nausea, vomiting, headache and diarrhoea.

Benign Intracranial Hypertension

This comprises headache and papilloedema, without evidence of a mass lesion or hydrocephalus, but occasionally with slit-like ventricles on CT scan, and a CSF pressure usually of 250–500 mmH_2O. It may respond to weight reduction, salt restriction, or single or repeated lumbar puncture (daily at first and then every third day, removing 20–30 ml CSF until the pressure is below 180 mmH_2O). Diuretics, acetazolamide 250 mg three times daily, or oral glycerol 15–60 mg four times daily, are of limited value. Patients who do not respond may need prednisolone 60 mg daily, which usually relieves symptoms in a few days.

Post-Lumbar Puncture Headache

The traditional remedies are hydration, bed rest and analgesics, such as indomethacin 25–75 mg daily, or codeine phosphate 30–60 mg 3- to 4-hourly. Many anaesthetists, but few neurologists, recommend an epidermal patch with autologous blood.

Postconcussion and Other Headaches

Chronic anxiety, depression, dizziness and headache following head injury require repeated reassurance, benzodiazepines, antidepressants, beta-blockers and analgesics. The violent headache of acute subarachnoid haemorrhage may be alleviated to some extent by codeine phosphate 30–60 mg 3- to 4-hourly, with domperidone 10–20 mg p.o. if necessary to control nausea or vomiting. Cough headache is usually benign, but occasionally due to phaeochromocytoma or intracranial tumour. In the latter case, it is usual for cough to exacerbate rather than initiate the headache. Most sex headaches are benign, and not due to subarachnoid haemorrhage or brain stem infarction. Headache in hypertensive encephalopathy is associated with high diastolic blood pressure of above 120–140 mmHg, and usually responds within 48 h to effective hypotensive treatment. Dialysis headache may be due to migraine which is made worse by dialysis, or result from disequilibrium. Here the possibility of a subdural haemorrhage must be considered.

Thalamic Pain

The severe, persistent, unpleasant or intolerable pain in the hemiplegic limb after a stroke in the distribution of the posterior cerebral artery with thalamic infarction rarely responds to any analgesic. Sedatives (e.g. clonazepam 1 mg three times daily), antihistamines (e.g. cyproheptadine 4 mg three times daily), antidepressants (e.g. imipramine 75–150 mg daily), and phenothiazines (e.g. chlorpromazine 25–100 mg daily) sometimes give limited relief.

Pain Associated with Neurological Lesions

Brief, lancinating pains in multiple sclerosis, tabes dorsalis, and other spinal and nerve lesions occasionally respond to carbamazepine 200–600 mg daily or phenytoin 200–400 mg daily.

Phantom Limb Pain

Nerve injury can be followed by many different kinds of pain. Immediate effective analgesic and sedative treatment of painful peripheral nerve lesions may prevent the later development of painful phenomena in the limb. Phantom limb pain is one of the most terrible of these, and occurs in about 30% of patients after amputation, being permanent in 5%–10%. Sympathetic ganglia contribute to this pain in some way, but although sympathectomy will relieve the constant burning pain of causalgia, this operation does not produce lasting relief of phantom limb pain. In the presence of a tender stump, modification of the sensory input by anaesthetic block or intense stimulation occasionally gives pain relief.

The effects of drug treatment of phantom limb pains are usually disappointing, although regular analgesics (paracetamol 500 mg up to six times daily), combined with major tranquillisers (chlorpromazine 50–500 mg daily) may be partially successful. As with postherpetic neuralgia, continuous or intermittent transcutaneous electrical stimulation may make this kind of pain tolerable, as it may in patients with pain due to malignant disease, with nerve or root involvement. Cordotomy, either percutaneous or open, and dorsal root or column stimulation, are unsatisfactory in the long term. In all kinds of chronic pain, many different procedures will give limited short-term relief. These procedures include dorsal root blocks and the use of intrathecal ice-cold saline or morphine, as well as more radical procedures such as cordotomy, cingulotomy, thalamotomy, or even ablation of the sensory cortex. Acupuncture and hypnosis have little or no place in the relief of chronic severe pain, and there is probably a widespread disturbance of pain mechanisms in these patients, so that whatever level pain is attacked, it often returns.

Pain following brachial plexus avulsion injuries may be delayed, long-lasting and severe and may require any of the forms of treatment used for phantom limb pain. In addition, coagulation of the avulsed cervical dorsal root entry zones has been reported to give long-term pain relief in many cases refractory to other forms of treatment. If the patient is already addicted to narcotic analgesics, success is less likely.

Acute and Chronic Lumbar Pain

Acute lumbar pain is best managed by absolute rest, warm baths, benzodiazepines combined with aspirin, or if this is ineffective, indomethacin 50 mg twice daily (beware haematological and gastrointestinal side effects). A firm mattress with a bed board, local anaesthetic infiltration into trigger zones, and a firm corset may help. Chronic low back pain is best managed with analgesics, postural correction, exercises and a bed board. Traction serves to keep the patient in bed, but probably does little else. In acute lumbar disc herniation, surgery is indicated in patients with persistent severe pain, repeated attacks, or muscle wasting.

Symptom Control in Terminal Neurological Illness

Severe and overwhelming terminal pain is fortunately uncommon with cerebrovascular disease, brain tumours and degenerative disorders, although depression, fear, anxiety, mental isolation and other unrelieved symptoms will all increase the total pain experience. Paracetamol 1000 mg 4-hourly, or DXT, are particularly useful in bone pain, and useful adjuncts to stronger analgesics. Anti-inflammatory drugs, such as mefenamic acid 500 mg 6-hourly, help approximately half all patients with severe bone pain, and prednisolone 20–60 mg daily is as, or more, effective. Baclofen 30–80 mg daily will relieve painful flexor and extensor spasms in spinal cord disease. More severe pain requires morphine or diamorphine in a starting dose of 5–10 mg p.o. 4-hourly, if necessary potentiated by chlorpromazine 12.5–100 mg p.o. With diamorphine dosage may need to be increased every 2–3 days. Coma and respiratory depression due to morphine or diamorphine can be quickly reversed with naloxone 0.4–1.2 mg i.v., repeated every 10–15 min. Diamorphine 10–40 mg or even 60 mg p.o. given 4-hourly will usually control severe pain. If not, then half the oral dose may be given i.m., although the analgesic effect is shorter with parenteral than oral therapy.

The terminal stages of parkinsonism and motor neurone disease may be particularly distressing. Here, prednisolone 5 mg three times daily will produce an increase in appetite and sense of improved wellbeing. We not infrequently use morphine in small repeated doses in this situation as well. Anxiety and mental distress respond to benzodiazepine tranquillisers such as diazepam 2–10 mg twice daily, chlorpromazine, or morphine sulphate. If confusion predominates, haloperidol 1–5 mg p.o., or thioridazine 10–25 mg, may be combined with opiates, diazepam or chlormethiazole as necessary.

Further Reading

St. Christopher's Hospice (1976) Drug control of common symptoms. World Med 11 (8 September): 17–20
Lance JW (1981) Headache. Ann Neurol 10: 1–10

3 Prevention and Treatment of Cerebrovascular Disease

Nomenclature

TIA (transient ischaemic attack). Reversible ischaemic neurological defect with complete resolution within 24 h

RIND (reversible ischaemic neurological deficit). A focal neurological deficit of relatively rapid onset persisting for more than 24 h, but resolving completely within 3 weeks

PNS (partial nonprogressive stroke)

MID (multi-infarct dementia). Dementia attributable to separate episodes of cerebral infarction and/or ischaemia

Introduction

Prevention and Treatment of Stroke

After a major stroke, the brain will not grow again, and stroke prevention is much more important than treatment. Many of the risk factors for stroke have been identified, and every effort should be made to identify these and give the appropriate treatment before a calamitous stroke occurs. The greatest threat is the occurrence of a TIA, RIND or PNS. In attempts to prevent a major stroke, most of these patients are subjected to:

1. Antithrombotic drugs (fibrinolysins, anticoagulants, and platelet antiaggregants)
2. Extracranial arterial surgery

These procedures have also all been used after a major stroke has occurred, although there is little or no evidence that any of them is of much value here.

Epidemiology of Stroke

In many countries of the world where data is available, cerebrovascular disease is the third leading cause of death. However, throughout developed countries, there has been an overall decline in mortality in the last decade. Not only mortality from stroke, but also stroke occurrence, has declined. In some parts of the world, there has been an approximate, 5% per year, decline for both stroke deaths and those due to myocardial infarction. This is comparable to the dramatic reduction which antibiotics brought to the mortality figures from bacterial diseases 30 years ago. Thus, for example, in the period 1953–1959 in New Zealand, mortality from cerebrovascular disease declined in men and women respectively by 15% and 47%. This striking result may be due partly to the widespread improvement in community control of high blood pressure, although the decline in mortality in women commenced before the widespread use of antihypertensive therapy.

During the same period, there has been a striking reduction in deaths attributable to hypertension and to rheumatic heart disease. At the same time, there has been widespread awareness of the need to reduce cigarette smoking, prevent obesity, and, if not to become a marathon runner, at least to adopt a more active life style. These factors, together with the antibiotic prophylaxis of rheumatic fever, are probably much more important in the limitation of mortality due to stroke than the use of antithrombotic therapy, cholesterol-lowering drugs, or endarterectomy.

Risk Factors for Stroke

Many studies, particularly from Framingham, Massachusetts, have revealed the effects of a wide variety of both environmental and genetic factors on the development of cerebrovascular disease. The effect of different risk factors on stroke, and on heart disease, appears to be different. Thus, smoking and lack of exercise have a greater effect on the likelihood of developing myocardial infarction than of developing a stroke, whereas with hypertension, the converse is true.

The most important preventable or potentially treatable predictors of stroke that have been recognised from the Framingham experience are as follows:

1. Hypertension at any level above 160 mmHg systolic and 90 mmHg diastolic, in both males and females and at any age
2. Haematocrit above normal levels
3. Impaired cardiac function, especially atrial fibrillation with, but also without, rheumatic disease

4. Asymptomatic carotid bruits and stenosis

5. The occurrence of TIAs

6. Smoking

7. Diabetes (even perhaps a slightly abnormal glucose tolerance test); other metabolic factors including obesity; and nonatheromatous vascular disease

A discussion of separate aspects of stroke prevention follows.

Stroke Prevention

Hypertension and Stroke

Most if not all lacunar strokes occur in patients with inadequately treated hypertension. The incidence of this type of stroke has declined with better monitoring and treatment of hypertension in the community. In addition, nonaneurysmal cerebral haemorrhage is largely confined to hypertensive subjects, and the incidence of atherosclerotic thrombotic stroke is much higher in hypertensive than in nonhypertensive subjects.

A diastolic blood pressure of 100 mmHg or more, or systolic pressure of 160 mmHg or more (systolic blood pressures are much more variable than diastolic), is associated with an approximate 2-fold increase in risk of cerebral infarction in men, and a 2.5-fold risk in women, without previous stroke. In men, about one-third of all cerebral strokes are attributable to a systolic blood pressure of 150 mmHg or more, and one-quarter of all strokes to a diastolic blood pressure of 95 mmHg or more.

The single most important measure therefore in preventing stroke is effective control of hypertension, even at relatively low levels. This treatment needs to be combined with reduction in excess weight, eating less saturated fat and more unsaturated fat, and limitation of salt consumption.

Management of Hypertension (Table 3.1)

Mild to Moderate Hypertension

Step 1. A beta-blocker is probably the drug of first choice in young hypertensives without heart failure, bronchospasm or peripheral vascular disease. The choice of beta-blocker is determined by side effects as well as the therapeutic action, so that atenolol 100 mg once daily or metoprolol 100 mg twice daily may be better choices than propranolol or oxprenolol 40 mg given more frequently. (The latter are short-acting, although sustained-release preparations are available.) If intrinsic sympathomimetic activity is needed (e.g. in heart failure), then pindolol 5 mg two or three times daily (up to 45 mg) is available, and with renal impairment nadolol may be a good choice

because of increased renal perfusion. With poor glomerular function, the
longer-acting drugs are less suitable because of possible toxicity related to
reduced renal clearance (this is an indication for reduction of dosage or
increasing the dose interval).

Table 3.1. Drug choice and major actions in the management of moderate essential hypertension

Drug	Action
Thiazide diuretics	Reduce vascular response to noradrenaline
Loop diuretics	Deplete sodium and reduce blood volume
Vasodilators	Reduce systemic resistance
Ganglion blockers	Reduce autonomic drive to resistance vessels and the heart
α-Adrenergic blocking drugs	Reduce vasomotor response in resistance vessels
β-Adrenergic blocking drugs	Reduce sympathetic drive to the heart
Central α-agonists	Activate hypotensive reflexes

Labetalol (see below) is an alpha-blocker which controls blood pressure
well, and has few side effects, but may lead to tachyphylaxis.

A diuretic is commonly used alone in the elderly. However, thiazide
diuretics induce hypokalaemia. Other problems with diuretics include
impaired glucose tolerance, urate excretion, frequency of micturition and
hypercholesterolaemia, and dehydration in the elderly.

Loop diuretics such as frusemide or bumetanide have their place to play in
renal failure, when fluid overload may contribute to the hypertension. Large
doses may then be needed. A combination of a beta-blocker and thiazide
diuretic is sometimes considered as a first-line approach in the treatment of
hypertension, and has been exploited commercially, although it is preferable
to use one or other of the drugs separately in the first instance. Beta-blockers
alone are now being used more frequently in the elderly. (See Table 3.2 for
notes on the choice of beta-blocker.)

Table 3.2. Choice of β-adrenergic blocking drugs in the management of hypertension

Drug	Cardioselectivity	CNS penetration	Daily dosage in hypertension (mg)	$t_{1/2}$ (h)	First-pass hepatic metabolism (%)
Propranolol	0	+	60– 320	2–6	70
Oxprenolol	0	+	160– 480	1–2	40
Pindolol	0	+	5– 45	3–4	15
Metoprolol	+	Poor	200– 400	3–4	50
Atenolol	+	Poor	50– 100	6–9	
Labetalol	0[a]	Poor	300–2400	3–4	

[a] Labetalol also has some alpha-blocking action.

1. *Central or Peripheral Action.* Atenolol, nadolol and sotalol are water-soluble, and less likely to cause central actions than lipid-soluble compounds. There are β-receptors in the hypothalamus, basal ganglia, limbic system and cerebellum, and the central effect of lipid-soluble beta-blockers may partially account for reduction in anxiety and tremor, as well as sedation, sleep disturbance and nightmares. However, the antitremor effect, reduction in palpitations and sweating, caused by beta-blockers, is largely peripheral in origin.

2. *Selectivity.* Cardioselective beta-blockers inhibit the β_1-receptors of the heart, but have little effect on β_2-receptors in the bronchi, and may not block vasodilator β_2-receptors. Metoprolol, atenolol and acebutolol are cardioselective, and may cause less coldness of the extremities and less increase in bronchial resistance than propranolol. In practice, cardioselectivity diminishes at high doses, and all beta-blockers may precipitate dangerous asthma.

3. *Sympathomimetic Agonist Activity.* Some beta-blockers stimulate as well as block adrenergic receptors. Drugs with intrinsic partial agonist activity reduce the heart rate less than those without it. Oxprenolol, pindolol and acebutolol will stimulate β-adrenoceptors as well as block the effect of injected catecholamines. In practice this effect is of little importance in the treatment of hypertension, although pindolol may increase rather than reduce essential tremor.

4. *Duration of Action.* Since sustained-release preparations of beta-blockers are available, once-daily dosage is generally possible with many drugs. The plasma level can vary widely (by a factor of 20) for a given dose in normal people with propranolol and other beta-blockers.

Disadvantages of Beta-blockers. Beta-blockers may cause mild coldness of the extremities, muscle fatigue, sleep disturbance, limitation of exercise tolerance, and sedation. They should not be used in patients with uncontrolled heart failure, severe diabetes with frequent insulin hypoglycaemia, severe peripheral vascular disease or asthma. With chronic mild obstructive airway disease, metoprolol or atenolol is preferable to propranolol or oxprenolol, but cardioselectivity is relative, not absolute. Treatment of cardiovascular disease with beta-blockers should not be stopped abruptly, but the drug should be withdrawn slowly over several days.

Practolol, which was withdrawn a decade ago, caused an oculomucocutaneous syndrome, with conjunctival scarring, psoriasiform rash, and retroperitoneal fibrosis. Skin rashes and dry eyes with other β-receptor blocking drugs are uncommon, and usually resolve on drug withdrawal.

Beta-blocker overdosage with excessive bradycardia can be countered with atropine 1–2 mg i.v., followed if necessary with a β-receptor stimulant such as isoprenaline 25 μg i.v.

Step 2. It may be necessary to use drug combinations for good blood pressure control, and some form of vasodilator is increasingly popular. Hydralazine 25–30 mg daily gives both preload and afterload reduction. Prazosin (an alpha-1 blocker) 1–5 mg two to four times a day gives good afterload reduction.

The calcium channel blocker nifedipine 10–20 mg three times a day in capsule form, or in the long-acting tablet preparation of 20–40 mg twice daily, lowers blood pressure. Also an antianginal, it can be used alone as a first-line drug for hypertension, especially in those who cannot take a beta-blocker. Verapamil 40–120 mg three times a day has a similar use.

Step 3. Minoxidil 5–50 mg daily may be added if combinations of beta-blocker, vasodilators, calcium channel blockers and diuretics have not succeeded (hirsutes can be marked with this drug). α-Methyldopa 250–500 mg two to four times a day can be added, but has side effects of postural hypotension, depression and Coombs-positive haemolytic anaemia.

Ganglion blockers (such as guanethidine and clonidine) are now virtually never used in initiating treatment.

The serum angiotensin-converting enzyme inhibitor captopril has so far accrued the side effects of hyperkalaemia, neutropenia, worsening glomerular filtration rate (possibly with a renal artery stenosis) and, rarely, an interstitial nephritis, but undoubtedly can sometimes control blood pressure if steps 1–3 are not sufficient. It is not universally successful. Small doses must be introduced first, with a test dose of 5 or 12.5 mg given lying down. It can be used alone in doses of 12.5–50 mg three or four times a day orally, but is more effectively used with a diuretic.

The Hypertensive Emergency

Malignant hypertension in which severe hypertension is complicated by papilloedema and proteinuria should, if at all possible, be controlled by bed rest and oral preparations of beta-blockers, diuretics or calcium antagonists. Precipitous falls of blood pressure are as dangerous as the severe hypertension and may cause a stroke, myocardial infarction, or acute tubular necrosis and acute renal failure. In patients with malignant hypertension who present with hypertensive encephalopathy, and in whom oral agents do not greatly lower blood pressure, consideration should be given to the use of labetalol, hydralazine or sodium nitroprusside. These are all potent drugs.

Labetalol has both α- and β-receptor blocking activity. It causes vasodilatation without tachycardia and, unlike other beta-blockers, has an immediate hypotensive effect. It may be given i.v. for rapid control, labetalol 50 mg i.v. over 1 min repeated every 5 min until 200 mg has been given. Alternatively, slow infusion labetalol 2 mg/min will lower blood pressure for 4–6 h without tachycardia or increase in cardiac output.

Hydralazine is a useful addition to beta-blockers and thiazide diuretics. Given by slow i.v. injection, 20–40 mg over 2 h will lower blood pressure in a hypertensive crisis, but like diazoxide produces tachycardia, as well as fluid retention and a lupus erythematosus-like syndrome during long-term use with more than 200 mg daily.

Hypertension in Pregnancy

Essential hypertension in pregnancy can be safely and successfully treated by conventional doses of a beta-blocker, labetalol, methyldopa or hydralazine. A hypertensive or preeclamptic emergency associated with neurological symptoms can be treated with parenteral hydralazine, labetalol or sodium nitroprusside if oral medication is not effective.

Haematocrit and Stroke

There is a very close relationship between the O_2 content of arterial blood and cerebral blood flow. When the haemoglobin concentration increases, cerebral blood flow falls. Anaemia, by reducing the oxygen-carrying capacity of the blood, increases the flow requirement with cerebral arterioles at the dilatated end of their range of diameters and reduces the effectiveness of collateral supply. Polycythaemia increases the viscosity of blood and, in particular, reduces flow along collateral channels, with a reduced range of pressure over which autoregulation in the cerebral circulation is effective.

Both anaemia and polycythaemia therefore predispose to stroke, although the boundaries of optimum limits for normal haematocrit in men and women are not closely defined. Certainly in the presence of TIAs, Hb should be increased to 10 g/dl or more in anaemia, and reduced to 16–18 g/ dl or less in polycythaemia.

Stroke and Heart Disease

Heart disease and hypertension are the chief risk factors for both an initial and a second stroke. Cardiac abnormalities are very frequent in stroke patients, and usually reflect the presence of coexisting heart disease. However, acute stroke itself may lead to ventricular ectopic activity, heart block, and myocardial damage.

The risk of a heart attack after recovery from an acute stroke is even greater than the risk of a second stroke. Some studies have indicated that about 30% of TIA and other minor stroke victims will have a major stroke, or be dead of myocardial infarction, within 3 years of the onset of first TIA.

Embolising Heart Disease (Table 3.3)

Rheumatic valvular heart disease on the left side, recent myocardial infarct involving the endocardium of the left ventricle, and hearts with an artificial mitral or aortic valve are common sources of emboli. In these cases, as well as with mechanical prosthetic valves, lifelong anticoagulant treatment is necessary.

When such hearts start to embolise in spite of anticoagulants, the possibility of platelet thrombi forming on the valve is difficult to exclude, and antiplatelet treatment as well as anticoagulants then seems rational. When an embolic infarct arises as a result of rheumatic heart disease, lone atrial fibrillation or myocardial infarction, it is usual to anticoagulate the patient (see p. 36) in the hope of preventing further emboli, in spite of the occasional conversion of a pale embolic infarct to a haemorrhagic infarct, with a worse prognosis. Perhaps this possibility can be minimised by treating any hypertension first (after the acute phase), and then waiting 2–3 weeks for the infarct to mature before starting anticoagulants. The right decision depends on (a) the severity of the stroke—a major completed stroke speaking against anticoagulation—and (b) the likelihood of further embolism, as judged from cardiac investigation; for example, as to whether friable-looking thrombus is still present in the heart.

Table 3.3. Cardiac sources of emboli

Site	Pathology
Left atrium	Thrombus
	Myxoma
	Paradoxical embolus
Mitral valve	Rheumatic endocarditis
	Infective endocarditis
	Leaflet prolapse
	Mitral ring calcification
	Prosthetic valve
Left ventricle	Myocardial infarction
	Cardiomyopathy
	Left ventricular aneurysm
Aortic valve	Rheumatic endocarditis
	Infective endocarditis
	Bicuspid valve
	Calcified valve
	Prosthetic valve
	Syphilitic aortitis
Congenital heart disease	
Cardiac surgery	Air embolism
	Platelet/fibrin embolism

A variety of cardiac lesions, including cardiac myxoma, postmyocardial infarction, akinetic segments, prolapsing mitral valve, mitral ring calcification, as well as classical mural thrombi, following infarction and mitral stenosis of rheumatic origin, produce TIAs. Bacterial endocarditis occurs in 3% of patients with mitral valve prolapse, and there is no doubt that cerebral infarction is more common in people with prolapsed valves than in the general population, particularly in young patients. Most of these lesions can be identified readily with cardiac imaging techniques. However, the yield of clinically useful information from echocardiography is low, even when cerebral emboli from a cardiac source are suspected on clinical or radiographic grounds, and it is rare for echo cardiography to give definite support for the use of anticoagulants.

Nonembolic TIAs

In the last decade, a number of noncardiac disorders have been identified which produce typical TIA symptoms. On the whole, these occur in young individuals not expected to have severe atheroma, although the clinical presentation may be indistinguishable. Fibromuscular dysplasia and spontaneous dissection are not uncommon in the extracranial course of the major cerebral arteries.

Carotid Artery Disease, Stenosis and Bruits

Atherosclerosis affecting the internal carotid artery near its origin is the most common disease process, but a number of other different diseases affect the artery at different points in its course from the thorax to the brain, and may cause symptoms of cerebral ischaemia. These include arteritis, dissection, dysplasia, kinking and looping, and trauma. Similar diseases affect the vertebral artery in the neck. Terminal portions of the internal carotid artery and the circle of Willis passing through the subarachnoid space may be affected by chronic inflammatory or granulomatous lesions here. Distal to the occlusion, there may be marked dilatation of intracerebral arteries to give a moyamoya pattern.

Fibromuscular dysplasia most commonly affects the middle third of the internal carotid artery in females. Although usually asymptomatic, some patients have transient visual or ischaemic episodes, probably due to thromboembolism. Platelet antiaggregants such as aspirin, rather than surgical treatment, should be used.

Injury to the carotid or vertebral arteries, either penetrating or non-penetrating, sometimes causes stroke, particularly in young people. Stroke due to vertebral artery damage follows a variety of neck movements, even yoga exercise, and in some patients repeated trauma over months or years, leading to local thrombus formation over an area of intimal damage, appears to be responsible for embolism, dissection or occlusive thrombosis. A specific event, for example neck turning whilst parking a car, occasionally seems to precipitate a stroke. Strangulation and stab wounds, as well as forcible lateral or backward stretching of the neck, as in a motorcycle injury, may be followed after a latent period of some hours by a sudden hemiparesis.

The management of patients with carotid trauma presents many difficulties. Medical treatment with anticoagulants is usually preferable to exploration and removal of thrombosis from the internal carotid artery in the neck.

Carotid looping and kinking in adults usually results from lengthening of the vessel owing to atherosclerosis and hypertension. This may be associated with TIAs, and very occasionally resection of the redundant loop leads to a dramatic cure.

Carotid or vertebral artery dissection is usually spontaneous, associated with fibromuscular dysplasia, Marfan's syndrome, or pseudoxanthoma elasticum. Other cases are traumatic. The condition is not necessarily fatal, and frequently resolves spontaneously. Angiography shows a tapered vessel and a very attenuated segment up to the skull base.

The usual cause of carotid artery disease is atherosclerosis. Atheroma begins as a subintimal fatty deposition at sites of increased trauma, areas of turbulence, arterial bifurcations, or with sudden changes in arterial calibre. The incidence of carotid atheroma is increased in hypertension. The carotid bifurcation is the most common site for atheroma in the carotid tree, and stenosis of the internal carotid near its origin is a frequent cause of both carotid occlusion and cerebral embolism. Carotid artery disease may be symptomless, or cause cerebral ischaemia, due to embolism or as a result of generalised insufficiency in the collateral blood supply, with occlusion of other extracranial arteries or an incomplete circle of Willis. There are many reports of symptomless patients with three of the four vessels completely occluded, and resting cerebral blood flow measurements in these patients have been normal. When symptomatic, focal carotid atherosclerosis is best treated medically, not surgically (see p. 49).

Diagnosis of Carotid Artery Disease

The clinical diagnosis of carotid artery disease is often made by finding a bruit. Subsequent management presents many difficulties. Carotid arteriography is the traditional method for definitively demonstrating carotid stenosis, with views in two planes, but it is sometimes difficult to distinguish a tight stenosis from occlusion, and puncturing a diseased carotid artery occasionally causes embolism or occlusion. Pulsed Doppler ultrasound can detect stenosis and distinguish between internal carotid occlusion and a very tight stenosis, as well as between a normal carotid and one with a small but ulcerated plaque which may be embolising. Digital vascular imaging, although with less risk than direct carotid arteriography, is not entirely without risk, and techniques at present available do not always adequately define the intracerebral circulation. CT scanning is of help in the investigation of TIAs when cerebral infarction or ventricular irregularity is recognised, as well as in those cases where TIAs are caused by cerebral tumour or aneurysm.

Management of Carotid Artery Disease

Table 3.4 summarises the management of the different forms of carotid artery disease.

Table 3.4. Management of carotid artery disease

Disease	Management
Carotid atherosclerosis	Platelet antiaggregants rather than surgery
Fibromuscular dysplasia	Platelet antiaggregants (mechanical dilatation may induce dissection)
Carotid artery trauma	Anticoagulants rather than surgical removal of thrombus; if emboli recur, consider internal carotid ligation
Carotid looping and kinking	Consider resection of redundant loop in adults
Carotid artery dissection	None
Carotid inflammatory disease	Corticosteroids, immunosuppressive drugs

Transient Ischaemic Attacks

Not all brief focal neurological symptoms in either the old or the young are TIAs. A diagnosis of ischaemic origin symptoms can not be substantiated unless there is definite evidence of sensory, motor or brain stem involvement, with symptoms of amaurosis fugax, double vision, dysphasia, true vertigo, or limb weakness. Vague complaints such as dizziness, light-headedness, drop attacks, memory disturbances and slurring of speech, do not necessarily indicate that a TIA has occurred. In addition, conditions that may mimic TIAs, such as migraine, partial epilepsy, Meniere's syndrome, or even attacks of acute glaucoma, must be distinguished. This distinction is impossible on history alone in at least a quarter of all patients.

If the symptomatology of TIA can be critically appraised, it is necessary to identify the part of the cerebral circulation involved, whether carotid or vertebrobasilar. Unless clear distinguishing features occur, the presentation may be misleading. It is most important to recognise that not all typical TIA symptoms are due to embolism. An increasing variety of disorders has been identified which produces similar symptoms. In addition to those conditions discussed on p. 32, these include cerebrovascular spasm in accelerated hypertension, anaemia, polycythaemia and hypotensive episodes. In about 5% of patients suffering from TIAs, the symptoms can be reproduced by inducing hypotension on a tilt-table, suggesting watershed ischaemia.

Most TIAs are probably due to the presence of a cardiac or vascular source of emboli. Successive emboli from the same source often produce identical attacks, since lamination of arterial blood flow makes it likely that successive emboli will take the same route; and also most possible sites of embolic lodgement are not end-artery sites. Many emboli move on or break up after temporarily lodging at a point where the collateral circulation is poor. Many cerebral emboli do not cause symptoms. In multi-infarct disease, the number of infarcts observed at post mortem or on CT scan is usually much greater than the number of clinical stroke episodes.

TIAs are harbingers of stroke, although some studies have indicated that only one stroke in eight or nine will be preceded by TIA. Nevertheless, 40%

of patients with TIA have proceeded to stroke in the Framingham prospective study. Other studies have indicated that about 30% of TIA and RIND patients will have a stroke or be dead of myocardial infarction within 3 years of the onset of TIA symptoms.

Strategies Utilised to Reduce the Threat of Stroke Following TIA

Following TIA, RIND or PNS, many patients are submitted to antithrombotic therapy (fibrinolysins, anticoagulants and platelet antiaggregants), as well as extracranial arterial surgery. Anticoagulants will prevent venous but not arterial thrombosis. Antiplatelet drugs will not prevent venous thromboembolism, but may inhibit thrombosis in the arterial circulation, where thrombi are formed by platelet aggregation. Because of major problems with haemorrhage, most TIA or RIND patients, where atherothrombosis is judged to be the pathogenesis, are treated by antiaggregants as the first line of defence.

Anticoagulants

Anticoagulants have never been properly assessed in stroke-risk patients. In a number of studies, the occurrence of TIAs in patients given anticoagulants is diminished, but stroke not prevented, and morbidity and mortality not decreased. Antiplatelet drugs, not anticoagulants, should be the first line of defence against thrombosis in the arterial circulation.

There are a number of pathological mechanisms for TIA and PNS where it is reasonable to give heparin or coumarin derivatives (Table 3.5). Many are heart disorders, and basically all are circumstances where thrombogenesis from triggering of the coagulation cascade may be postulated.

In most conditions shown in Table 3.5, anticoagulants should be given for periods of time varying from a few weeks to 3–4 months. Treatment may prevent the repeated formation and embolism of thrombus on an ulcerated plaque, and give the vascular endothelium a chance to recover the ulcer. Removing an embolising plaque by carotid endarterectomy improves the angiogram, but leaves the vessel temporarily denuded of endothelium, so a period of anticoagulants is rational. Anticoagulant withdrawal should be gradual because of the supposed but controversial rebound effect after coumarin withdrawal. Anticoagulants should be continued indefinitely where there is a known continuing source of emboli such as atrial fibrillation.

Heparin. Heparin is a mucopolysaccharide originally discovered by McLean in 1916 whilst a medical student at Johns Hopkins. Heparin was found in animal tissues, although it cannot be detected in the circulating blood. Heparin prevents blood clotting in vitro as well as in vivo, 1 unit in vitro being equivalent to 120 units in vivo. Heparin is precipitated by acid, and is not active orally or absorbed through the gastrointestinal tract. Given intravenously, it has an immediate anticoagulant effect, and inhibits the

Table 3.5. Empirical recommendations for anticoagulant usage (Barnett 1984)

---

*1. Recent myocardial infarction—large, septal, with heart failure or atrial fibrillation, or with clinical evidence of cerebral or retinal ischaemia; or with echocardiogram evidence of a thrombus

*2. Previous myocardial infarction, with akinetic segment and cerebral and retinal ischaemic events

*3. Mitral stenosis with or without atrial fibrillation

*4. Prosthetic heart valve

*5. Atrial fibrillation for other reasons, with any evidence of cerebral or systemic emboli

6. Progressing stroke under observation, decline occurring over several hours

7. Thrombus detectable in stenosed cerebral artery

**8. Recognised disorders of coagulation mechanisms in the presence of retinal or cerebral ischaemia

9. Failure of platelet antiaggregants to prevent a great many TIAs, more prolonged episodes (RIND) or PNS in the following conditions:
    (a) atherothrombotic mechanisms with emboli attributed to them
    (b) prolapsing mitral valve
    (c) mitral ring calcification
    (d) fibromuscular dysplasia or arterial dissections

---

* Duration of therapy indefinite in these conditions.
** See p. 39 for treatment of disseminated intravascular coagulation.

conversion of prothrombin to thrombin dependent on the presence of an IgA cofactor, antithrombin III. Heparin also reduces the concentration of triglycerides in plasma.

The effects of heparin are short-lived ($t_{1/2}$=90 min). Because of this, and if the drug is given infrequently, the anticoagulant effect is erratic. Heparin should therefore be given:

1. Ideally by infusion pump rather than drip. Heparin should be given in saline, not dextrose, which may reduce the anticoagulant effect, with a loading dose of 5000 units and 1500 units hourly (40 000 units over 24 h)

2. Intermittent i.v. therapy 10 000 units 6-hourly

3. Low-dose heparin s.c. 5000 units 12-hourly to prevent postoperative, postpartum, postmyocardial infarction thrombosis

4. Heparin i.m. produces irregular absorption and local haematoma, and should not be used

Regimes 1 and 2, but not 3 require long-term laboratory monitoring, although if heparin is given intermittently for 48 h at the start of oral anticoagulant therapy, 3- to 6-hourly monitoring is unnecessary. Heparin affects all stages of anticoagulation, and prolongs the clotting time, the prothrombin time and the thrombin–fibrinogen reaction. Plasma heparin levels are of no clinical value, since the drug effect is indicated by the clotting screen.

Heparin is not protein-bound, is concentrated in blood vessel endothelium, and is rapidly and largely metabolised by the liver. The anticoagulant effect of heparin is increased by antiplatelet drugs, aspirin, dipyridamole and sulphinpyrazone. Bleeding due to heparin overdosage may be reversed with protamine sulphate 1% solution, 1 mg neutralising 100 units heparin, maximum dose 50 mg.

Oral Anticoagulants. Warfarin is derived from coumarin, phenindione from indan 1:3 dione. Both prevent liver synthesis of prothrombin, factors VII, IX and X, by competitive inhibition of vitamin K. The anticoagulant effect takes 36–48 h to develop, and lasts for 1–4 days after drug withdrawal. The oral anticoagulant dose should be adjusted to prolong the prothrombin time to 2–4 times normal values. Prothrombin time should be measured daily for the first 4 days, then weekly, and then monthly when stable dosage has been established. Plasma drug levels are not of clinical value. Alcohol interferes with the metabolism of warfarin.

Warfarin absorption from the alimentary tract is nearly complete, and 97% of warfarin is bound to albumin in plasma. The basal pattern of metabolism is inherited, with a similar $t_{1/2}$ in identical, but not in nonidentical twins.

The side effects of warfarin and phenindione are different. Warfarin (starting dose 20 mg, maintenance dose range 2–20 mg daily) may cause skin necrosis, alopecia, abortion, but less sensitivity reactions than phenindione (200 mg on first day, 100 mg second day, maintenance 50–150 mg daily), which causes sensitivity reactions, rash, fever, leucopenia, agranulocytosis, renal and hepatic damage, and blocks iodine uptake by the thyroid. Phenindione metabolites produced by hydroxylation in hepatic microsomes may cause pink urine.

Unlike heparin, oral anticoagulants cross the placenta and enter milk. They may be teratogenic, and should not be given in the first trimester or the last weeks of pregnancy. Old people are more sensitive to the anticoagulant effect than young people.

Haemorrhage may require blood transfusion or phytomenadione (vitamin K_1) 20 mg i.v. This takes 6–12 h to act, and prevents oral anticoagulants acting for several days.

The following contraindications to oral anticoagulants should be noted:

1. Bleeding from any site
2. Potential bleeding, e.g. gastric ulcer
3. Haemorrhagic diathesis
4. Dissecting aneurysm
5. CNS surgery
6. Hypertension with diastolic blood pressure over 100 mmHg
7. Liver disease
8. Severe diabetes
9. Renal insufficiency

10. Poor cooperation, low intelligence, old age
11. Alcoholism

Occasionally, anticoagulants convert an ischaemic to haemorrhagic infarct. The interactions of oral anticoagulants with other drugs are summarised in Table 3.6.

Table 3.6. Drug interactions with oral anticoagulants

Effect	Drug
A. *Enhancement*	
Inhibition of hepatic metabolism	Phenylbutazone
	Alcohol
	Reserpine
Displacement from plasma binding	Aspirin
	Sulphonamides
	Phenytoin
Reduced vitamin K synthesis or absorption	Broad-spectrum antibiotics
	Liquid paraffin
B. *Reduction*	
Induction of hepatic drug-metabolising enzymes	Carbamazepine
	Phenytoin
	Barbiturates
	Haloperidol

Anticoagulants and Disseminated Intravascular Coagulation. Disseminated intravascular coagulation, DIC, has been recognised increasingly over the last decade. The condition is associated with a number of localised or generalised stimuli to clotting, including infection and neoplasms as well as liver failure. Laboratory criteria for DIC are a prolonged prothrombin time, thrombocytopenia and hypofibrinogenaemia. It is not always clear whether episodic cerebral dysfunction associated with DIC is due to vascular or metabolic disease and, overall, cerebral bleeding or infarction is uncommon. Patients with a malignancy and the clinical presentation of a large vessel stroke are likely to have DIC and nonbacterial thrombotic endocarditis. Recorded cerebrovascular consequences of DIC are large vessel occlusion, subarachnoid haemorrhage, and multiple cortical and brain stem haemorrhages and infarction. Some of these patients are at risk of haemorrhagic complications, and the results of heparin therapy for DIC are sometimes deleterious, not favourable.

Platelet Antiaggregants

Several drugs reduce platelet adhesiveness, by acetylation of platelet membrane proteins, and by prostaglandin inhibition. These drugs may have an additive effect, although a synergistic action of the most commonly used combination, aspirin and dipyridamole, has not been demonstrated clinically.

Aspirin is probably effective, at least in men, in reducing the incidence of stroke, or stroke death, or stroke and sudden death. The best dose is unclear. Some laboratory evidence suggests that a very small dose (e.g. 60 mg daily) is needed. However, most patients are given between 300 mg and 1 g daily. Clofibrate, sulphinpyrazone and dipyridamole have yet to be shown to be beneficial, alone or in combination, in stroke prevention. Dipyridamole has been shown in other clinical trials to improve patency of bypass grafts in coronary artery surgery, and may reduce embolism from prosthetic heart valves. The suggested benefit from aspirin is considerable, with a 50% reduction in stroke or sudden death. Aspirin has not been shown to reduce recurrence rate in patients with myocardial infarction, but alone or combined with dipyridamole there is a substantial reduction in the number of strokes following myocardial infarction, as compared with placebo.

Aspirin, 300 mg 8-hourly, inhibits platelet release, and will prolong bleeding time for 5 days. Aspirin inhibits platelet cyclo-oxygenase, and stops the production of cyclic endoperoxides and thromboxane A_2.

Sulphinpyrazone 200 mg 8-hourly is a strong organic acid, well absorbed from the gut, 95% plasma-bound, mostly excreted unchanged in the urine, and used as an uricosuric drug in the treatment of gout. It is a weak competitive inhibitor of platelet prostaglandin synthesis, and may prevent platelets sticking to blood vessel walls. Sulphinpyrazone can cause hypersensitivity, rashes and fever, gastrointestinal irritation, and possibly depress haemopoiesis. There is no evidence that sulphinpyrazone reduces the frequency of amaurosis fugax or other cerebrovascular accidents.

Dipyridamole 400 mg daily was originally used as a coronary vasodilator, although this action is doubtful. However, the drug does cause vasodilation and hypotension. It modifies platelet function by inhibiting phospho-diesterase and by stimulation of adenylate cyclase. The simultaneous use of aspirin (which decreases prostacyclin, and thus platelet cAMP) will prevent this effect. Dipyridamole in high concentration in vitro inhibits platelet release and aggregation. In low dosages in vivo (50–400 mg daily) dipyridamole has little demonstrable effect in preventing transient ischaemic attacks or improving cerebrovascular disease. It may cause mild nausea, headache, vomiting, and diarrhoea, as well as hypotension.

Smoking and Stroke

The number of cigarettes smoked, and the amount of tobacco in each cigarette, have declined in both America and western Europe in the last 20 years. There is good evidence that smoking is a risk factor for stroke, and the decline in the tobacco habit must account for some of the surprising decrease in stroke and heart disease over the last 20 years.

Diabetes, Other Metabolic Disorders and Nonatheromatous Vascular Disease

The association of diabetes mellitus and stroke is well recognised. Stroke is more frequent, and cerebral damage more severe, in diabetics than in nondiabetics. When ischaemia affects the brain, with high levels of carbohydrate, it produces greater neurological damage than with low carbohydrate levels. Careful control of blood sugar in diabetics should reduce the risk of stroke.

Minor degrees of hyperglycaemia, not uncommonly, precede a stroke, as determined by plasma levels of glycosylated haemoglobin. These levels reflect glycaemic levels for the previous 1–3 months, and are often found to be high, comparable to levels in diabetic patients, when measured following a stroke.

Familial and acquired hypercholesterolaemia, like diabetes and hypertension, accelerate the development of atheroma at the normal vulnerable points. Effective treatment of hypercholesterolaemia with diet and cholestyramine, like effective treatment of diabetes and hypertension, reduces the incidence of stroke. However, the same procedures have not been shown to reduce stroke incidence in subjects with normal blood lipids.

Hypotension and Stroke

With cerebral vessels of normal reactivity, cerebral blood flow is kept constant down to an arterial pressure of 50 mmHg or less. Cerebral arterioles dilate in response to increased pCO_2, decreased pO_2, or decreased pH. However, collateral blood supply becomes less effective in the hypotensive range; the pressure difference along the collaterals falls, and so does the flow. Owing to the reduced capacity for autoregulation in cerebrovascular disease, the blood pressure may have to be maintained within narrower limits than normal. Increased ischaemia or infarction in brain areas where blood flow autoregulation is impaired, can follow moderate hypotension. Volume expansion, induced hypertension, and vasodilators such as nitroprusside, used in conjunction with vasopressors, may prevent deterioration with progressive ischaemic symptoms and hypotension following stroke.

Sickle Cell Disease

Cerebral infarcts can occur when small vessels become occluded with sickled cells. Endothelial proliferation and occasionally cerebral haemorrhage can also occur. No treatment is really effective, apart from frequent transfusion to keep HbS low for at least 6 months. This may reduce thrombotic episodes.

Temporal Arteritis (see also pp. 16, 190)

Prednisolone 30–60 mg daily causes rapid pain relief, reduction in ESR, and a lessening of polymyalgia,. brachiocervical symptoms, visual loss and other vascular episodes. The overall mortality in treated patients is similar to that in the general population. However, there are many problems with steroid treatment of temporal arteritis, with frequent complications, drug-related fatalities; and eventual cure is often never achieved. Conventional wisdom is that steroids must be given to prevent, in particular, ciliary artery thrombosis, as well as to relieve headache. It is usually possible to reduce prednisolone dosage to around 10 mg daily within 3 months of starting treatment. Alternate-day steroid therapy in this or lower dosage is often sufficient to prevent headache, and keep the ESR below 30–40 mm/h. Starting steroids does not necessarily affect the result of biopsy, providing this is done within 1 week.

Cerebral Vasculitis

Corticosteroid treatment of isolated angiitis of the central nervous system is not nearly so successful as treatment of temporal arteritis. Fortunately, isolated angiitis of small cerebral (sometimes spinal) vessels is very uncommon, best diagnosed by a study of the angiographic appearance, and with a high ESR in patients with multifocal neurological deficits. Although steroid treatment alone is not very effective, combined steroid–immunotherapy may prevent disease progression and further strokes. Cyclophosphamide (see p. 142), 2 mg/ kg, should be combined with prednisolone 60 mg daily, using the ESR as the best guide as to when to reduce or stop treatment.

Oral Contraceptives

In young women, the normally very low incidence of cerebral thrombosis was increased almost tenfold, and of haemorrhage twofold, on early, high-progesterone contraceptive pills. The danger of low-dose pills is much slighter, but migraine, thromboembolism, hypertension and TIAs are all good reasons for withholding or withdrawing oral contraceptives.

Cortical Thrombophlebitis

Cortical thrombophlebitis often results from middle ear infection, sinusitis, head injury, dehydration, ulcerative colitis, polycythaemia or pregnancy; raised intracranial pressure and focal epilepsy usually occur, and cerebral infarction may follow. The common organisms in septic cerebral sinus thrombosis are *Staphylococcus aureus*, streptococci and pneumococci. Antibiotics should therefore include methicillin or cloxacillin in high dosage.

Treatment Following Major Cerebral Ischaemia

All the measures described for stroke prevention have also been adopted after major ischaemia (Table 3.7), although usually with little or no benefit. Despite recent interest in regrowth of the damaged infant nervous system, functional recovery following major damage to the adult nervous system is usually very incomplete.

Table 3.7. Treatment of stroke

A. *Prevention*
   Hypertension
   Diabetes
   Smoking
   Hyperlipidaemia
   Polycythaemia
   Anaemia

B. *Prevention following TIA, RIND*
   As above, plus consider:
      Anticoagulants
      Antiplatelet drugs
      Vascular surgery in vertebral steal syndromes

C. *Established stroke*
   As for TIAs, after the acute phase, if either:
      1. The source of emboli threatens other cerebrovascular territories, or:
      2. The infarct is incomplete in its own territory
      3. Also treat:
         Hypertension (2 weeks after the acute stroke phase)
         Cerebral oedema (if present)
         Subcortical haematoma causing focal signs, with surgery

D. *Rehabilitation*
   Physiotherapy, mobilisation, prevention of contractures and protection of pressure areas
      Speech therapy
      Occupational therapy
      Treat depression

Cerebral Haemorrhage

Systemic hypertension is present in 80%–90% of intracerebral haemorrhage. About half of all patients presenting with subarachnoid haemorrhage are hypertensive. Hypertension is believed to be responsible for the formation of microaneurysms on intracerebral arteries by inducing hypertrophy, hyaline degeneration, and small ruptures in the medial coat (Charcot–Bouchard aneurysms). One of these microaneurysms then presumably ruptures and destroys itself. If the artery is very small, the bleed may split white matter fibre bundles and then stop (through arterial spasm provoked by the perivascular blood); the haematoma affects surrounding brain by local pressure and distortion. When a small haematoma of this sort is absorbed, there may be excellent recovery of function. At post mortem years later there may be only a thin pigmented line to mark its place.

If the rupture is of a larger intracerebral artery, the force of the haemorrhage does much more local damage, and the space-occupying haematoma may cause herniation of the cingulate gyrus under the falx or of the uncus through the tentorial hiatus, with consequent distortion and compression of the midbrain and brain stem, causing secondary haemorrhages and infarctions there. This turn of events is usually fatal, and the damage is done too rapidly for surgical evacuation of the haematoma to be helpful. Rupture of a haematoma into the subarachnoid space or into a ventricle is also usually fatal. Draining intracerebral haematomas to reduce intracranial pressure has not been found to be life-saving, although dense focal signs are occasionally relieved by removing a subcortical haematoma.

Brain Stem Haemorrhage

Haemorrhage into the brain stem arises through a similar mechanism, but the opportunity for fibre-splitting haematomas to form and resolve without leaving a permanent deficit is much less. It is therefore usual for small brain stem haemorrhages to result in a permanent disability, or at least in permanent neurological signs. Larger brain stem haemorrhages are rapidly fatal. Cerebellar haematomas distorting the brain stem without yet causing permanent damage to it may be surgically removed with benefit.

Subarachnoid Haemorrhage

Subarachnoid haemorrhage from a ruptured saccular aneurysm, or (less commonly) an arteriovenous malformation of the brain, is the next most frequent cerebrovascular disorder following cerebral embolism, atherosclerosis and hypertensive intracerebral haemorrhage. The most common type of aneurysm (berry aneurysm) arises as a result of a congenital defect in the arterial media, often at a bifurcation in the region of the circle of Willis. The four most common sites are the anterior and posterior communicating arteries, middle cerebral, and the intracranial part of the internal carotid. Haemorrhage often occurs into the brain substance, causing an intracerebral haematoma, as well as into the subarachnoid space. A haematoma can cause focal signs, raised intracranial pressure, and disturbances of consciousness, while blood in the CSF causes meningeal irritation, headache and neck stiffness. Blood collected round the affected artery often causes arterial spasm, and secondary cerebral infarction often occurs.

Focal signs arising acutely from such a haematoma or infarct are not necessarily an accurate guide to the site of an aneurysm. Subarachnoid haemorrhage is diagnosed from a history of sudden severe headache, occasionally arising during exertion, with neck stiffness which may be very severe, and often loss of consciousness, of variable duration. It is confirmed by CT scan or, if this is not available, by lumbar puncture which, if done early, will show uniform bloodstaining of CSF, with xanthochromia after the first day.

Symptomatic vasospasm, or delayed cerebral ischaemia, associated with arteriographic evidence of arterial constriction, is at present the most important cause of morbidity after acute subarachnoid haemorrhage. The development of vasospasm is directly correlated with the presence of thick blood clots in the basal subarachnoid cisterns. Vasospasm usually develops 4–12 days after subarachnoid haemorrhage with, typically, a gradual deterioration of the level of consciousness, accompanied by focal neurological deficits that are determined by the arterial territories involved. Hyponatraemia frequently occurs and may exacerbate the symptoms. It has been suggested by several neurosurgeons, particularly in Japan, that early operation with removal of as much blood as possible from the subarachnoid cisterns may prevent vasospasm, although early operation was abandoned years ago by most neurosurgeons. Volume expansion, together with elevation of the systemic blood pressure, and reduction of the intracranial pressure when elevated, are the only available effective therapies for symptomatic vasospasm. The reader is referred to the review by Heros et al. (1983).

There is controversy as regards the efficacy and safety of antifibrinolytic agents following subarachnoid haemorrhage. The synthetic antifibrinolysin, aminocaproic acid, is sometimes given to delay fibrinolysis of the clot at the site of arterial rupture. The rebleeding rate may decrease considerably with this therapy. However, antifibrinolytic agents have been thought to increase the severity of vasospasm.

Antidiuretic hormone (ADH) has been used in patients following subarachnoid haemorrhage, with excessive urine output, but most of these patients already have elevated levels of ADH, and hyponatraemia can be exacerbated under these circumstances. Correction of the electrolyte balance may reverse focal neurological deficits.

Cerebral Angiomas

Angiomas account for only one-tenth as many subarachnoid haemorrhages as aneurysms, and occur in younger patients. The natural history is more favourable than with aneurysms, because angiomas are usually superficial where they are unlikely to cause intracerebral haematoma; and spasm in them, if it occurs, may be beneficial rather than leading to infarction. On the other hand, large angiomas may be difficult or impossible to treat surgically.

Cerebral Infarction

Inadequate blood supply causing infarction of part of the brain can arise through arterial embolism, occlusion, cerebrovascular spasm or watershed ischaemia. These mechanisms by which infarction can occur are separate, although linked in practice by common pathological processes. The processes leading to cerebral ischaemia and infarction are considered later, but what about the treatment of the damaged tissue itself? Brain that has just been infarcted will usually be surrounded by ischaemic tissue, which may also be oedematous. In order to limit the size of the infarct, it is desirable to increase blood flow through the ischaemic area. However, restoring blood flow through infarcted brain is likely to do a lot of harm, for two reasons:

1. A bloodless infarct may be converted into a haemorrhagic infarct, increasing space occupation.
2. The vessels in the infarcted area lose their autoregulation, and would carry an undue amount of blood, diverting blood away from the ischaemic surroundings.

It may therefore be helpful to treat focal oedema around an infarct using osmotic diuretics or steroids, but it is seldom beneficial to remove clot or embolus from an end-artery following infarction of its territory.

Cerebral Embolism

Emboli may come from the heart, particularly in rheumatic valvular disease with fibrillation, or from prosthetic valves. Emboli can also arise from mural thrombi following myocardial infarction; and infected emboli from vegetations occur in subacute bacterial endocarditis. More commonly, however, cerebral emboli arise from atheromatous plaques in the arterial tree, particularly in the region of the carotid bifurcation.

In order to produce symptoms of acute localised ischaemia, an embolus must lodge at a site where collateral supply to the territory is inadequate (end-artery); various events may then follow. First, the embolus may break up and pass distally to smaller vessels whose collateral communications are adequate, relieving the ischaemia. The embolus fragments subsequently lyse. Second, the ischaemic stimulus may provoke dilatation of the obstructed vessel (allowing distal movement of the embolus), or of collateral vessels (improving the collateral circulation), so relieving the ischaemia, but perhaps causing headache. Third, the embolus may remain in position, resulting in localised infarction of the acutely ischaemic area. Anterograde or retrograde propagation of thrombus in the vessel to the nearest branch does not alter the immediate situation, although it may make recanalisation more difficult. However, arterial thrombosis following embolism may extend distally or occasionally proximally past a branch or bifurcation so as to increase the ischaemic territory. Some deep penetrating vessels supply areas that lack collateral supply and are therefore particularly vulnerable to embolic damage, whereas the superficial circumferential vessels have numerous leptomeningeal connections.

Progressive Stroke

When progressive stroke occurs in a hypertensive crisis, the treatment is that of hypertension. Cerebral oedema, if present, is life-threatening, and can be treated with glycerol or mannitol; steroids are ineffective.

In nonhypertensive progressive stroke, the patient is anticoagulated, unless the CT scan shows intracerebral or subarachnoid blood. Hypothermia, anaesthesia, oxygenation and hyperbaric oxygen have been shown to be ineffective.

Treatment of Established Stroke

Attention to airway, pressure areas, bladder and nutrition is required, with physiotherapy to prevent chest infection and limb contractures. A hypertensive response to acute stroke is common, so hypertension first discovered following an acute stroke is not treated (unless severe, i.e. diastolic pressure sustained above 110 mmHg) for the first 2–3 days; remember the loss of autoregulation in the ischaemic zone. Cardiac failure or myocardial infarction may require treatment in their own right.

Cerebral Oedema in Stroke

Cerebral infarcts, particularly if large, often become surrounded by an area of oedema. The development of oedema may be suggested by the onset of drowsiness, failure of conjugate gaze towards the hemiplegic side, and an increase in weakness. Postinfarction oedema does not respond to steroids, but does respond to frusemide, glycerol or mannitol. Whether diuretics save life or reduce eventual disability is controversial; they probably do, provided they are given at the right time, and only to the patients who actually do have oedema.

Depression Following Stroke

Following an established stroke, many patients remain severely depressed for the rest of their lives, and antidepressant drug treatment is a vital part of stroke rehabilitation.

Watershed Ischaemia

Blood flow measurements in the healthy brain do not show a lesser perfusion of brain tissue at the border between the territories of two main arteries. It might be thought that tissue at such a watershed would be particularly protected against occlusion of either major vessel by virtue of its alternative blood supply. So when and why do watershed lesions occur?

Watershed infarction occurs: (a) in hypertensive encephalopathy; and (b) following episodes of prolonged hypotension or anoxia (for example anaesthetic accidents, or coma). In hypertensive encephalopathy, the patchy or diffuse vascular spasm present predominantly affects blood flow to the periphery of a vascular territory, as the arteriolar segments are longer.

In a normal brain, acute hypotension causes symptoms of watershed ischaemia (e.g. visual field constriction), followed by fainting. The change of posture restores blood flow and no damage is done. Prolonged hypotension or anoxia (as in anaesthetic accidents) can cause watershed infarcts. A degree of hypotension that fails to cause ischaemia in normal brain may lead to ischaemic damage: (a) in a brain whose primary supply is impaired and which is relying on a collateral supply; or (b) in a hypertensive brain whose arterioles are thickened, so that they cannot dilate fully. A collateral supply arises by anoxia-induced vasodilatation, and the dilated collaterals are incapable of dilating further in response to hypotension. Anaemia or polycythaemia may further impair the effectiveness of collateral supply for reasons given on p. 31.

Cerebrovascular Disease and Dementia

About 7% of all people over the age of 65 are demented, with impaired memory, intellect, personality, and disordered behaviour. Alzheimer's disease is the usual cause, but 10%–25% of elderly subjects have a cerebrovascular cause for their dementia. The common basis for the development of cerebrovascular dementia is multiple small infarcts, sometimes accompanied by watershed territory damage and often, if not always, in the presence of heart disease. Infarcts can be either embolic, often with a cardiac source, or result from hypertension, with the formation and rupture of multiple Charcot – Bouchard microaneurysms in cerebral penetrating vessels. It is important to separate patients with these types of MID from the majority with parenchymal degenerations such as Alzheimer's disease, since in the vascular group the hypertension or source of emboli should be treated in order to prevent progression of the dementia. However, clinical distinction is sometimes difficult. Points favouring a cerebrovascular cause of dementia are said to include hypertension, an abrupt stepwise history, periods of improvement, a history of strokes, focal neurological symptoms or signs, nocturnal confusion, depression, somatic complaints, emotional incontinence, and evidence of vascular disease elsewhere. None of these points is totally reliable; however, MID can be confirmed by CT scan, when this reveals a multitude of infarcts. Ventricular irregularity suggests MID as a cause for dementia. The progression of cerebrovascular disease with dementia can sometimes be halted by the treatment of hypertension, heart disease, and cardiac arrhythmias, which sometimes occur unrecognised during sleep.

Hydergine and Cerebral Vasodilators

Drug treatment for many different aspects of dementia, whether due to MID or Alzheimer's disease, is very unsatisfactory. Drugs used in the last decade to alter memory have included codeine, endorphins, phosphodiesterase inhibitors, benzodiazepines, central stimulant drugs, colchicine, vinblastine, choline, lecithin and ADH. Despite the demonstration that impairment of cognitive function in senile dementia (Alzheimer's type) is accompanied by impairment of cholinergic function, no effective rational treatment for Alzheimer's disease has been developed. Direct measurement of regional oxygen extraction by PET scanning has shown that chronic ischaemia has little role in the development of MID. Despite these negative findings, ergot drugs, which may alter cerebral metabolism or blood flow, so-called cerebral vasodilators, and choline and cholinergic drugs are widely used in parts of Europe, but not in the United Kingdom, in the treatment of senile or vascular dementia, despite widespread disbelief as to their effect.

Isoxsuprine, cyclandelate and naftidrofuryl oxalate have no role in the management of cerebrovascular disease. There is little doubt that Hydergine, the best studied and most reviewed of ergot derivatives in dementia, will cause improvement in mood and in some psychological tests, as well as in hypotension and sedation in old people, but rarely any worthwhile sustained benefit. Despite this, amongst Medicaid-aided elderly patients in California, Hydergine is second only to thioridazine in terms of drug expenditure amongst the institutionalised population.

Artery Surgery for Stroke

Asymptomatic Bruits

The risk of stroke is greater with a bruit or asymptomatic carotid stenosis than without these conditions, although the stroke may be on the opposite side or in posterior circulation. The temptation to do a carotid endarterectomy in asymptomatic cases once such a lesion is identified by noninvasive studies can be high, since it is argued that operation will reduce the risk of stroke. This temptation should be resisted. Even in the most skilled hands, the risks of angiography followed by endarterectomy exceed the risk of ipsilateral stroke.

Should asymptomatic carotid artery disease be surgically relieved before major abdominal, heart or aortic surgery? There are no convincing studies to help decide this question. There is no doubt that these patients are at risk of cerebral infarction during a period of perioperative hypotension, but in most centres in the world there seems little doubt that the arterial lesion is best left well alone.

Stenosis at the origin of one vertebral artery should not be an indication for operation unless the opposite vertebral artery is hypoplastic or there are osteophytes on the margins of the cervical vertebrae which impinge on the artery and its bony canal. More often than vertebral surgery, surgical removal of concomitant carotid lesions is an effective method of alleviating posterior circulation TIAs.

Surgical bypass operations, when the great vessels from the aorta are occluded, are of definite value, and may restore normal brain and retinal perfusion when this is reduced by focal or general atherosclerosis or nonspecific inflammatory disorder (Takayasu's arteritis) in oriental patients.

Superficial temporal–middle cerebral artery anastomosis has been practised since Yasargil described the operation in 1967, in an attempt at cerebral revascularisation following occlusion of the internal carotid artery and its branches. Recent studies have shown conclusively that in most subjects the procedure is of no value. Likewise, the benefit from omental grafting, from the abdomen to the meninges, either as a pedicle graft or free graft, as recently practised for stroke victims in China, has not been proven.

References and Further Reading

Barnett HJ (1984) Prevention of strokes. In: Callaghan N, Galvin R (eds) Recent research in neurology. Pitman, London, pp 77–84

Heros RC, Zervas NT, Varsos V (1983) Cerebral vasospasm after subarachnoid haemorrhage: an update. Ann Neurol 14: 599–608

Ross Russell RW (ed) (1983) Vascular disease of the central nervous system, 2nd edn. Churchill Livingstone, London

Reneman RS, Hoecks APG (1982) Doppler ultrasound in the diagnosis of cerebrovascular disease. Wiley, Chichester

4 Epilepsy

Epilepsy can be severely disruptive of life at home and at work. The medical management of epileptic seizures, whether single or recurrent, therefore involves much more than deciding to start anticonvulsant drug treatment. It includes:

1. Determining the cause and eliminating it (if possible)
2. Giving appropriate advice concerning the avoidance of fits, and the avoidance of injury or danger resulting from them
3. Treatment with anticonvulsant drugs, if possible with laboratory control
4. Genetic counselling
5. Occasionally surgery in drug-resistant focal, especially psychomotor, fits
6. Careful long-term follow-up
7. Deciding whether, when and how to withdraw drug treatment

Diagnosis and Choice of Treatment in Epilepsy

Table 4.1 classifies the main forms of epilepsy, and indicates the treatment of choice in each case. A careful history from the patient and if possible also from a parent or other witness is the best and often the only guide to diagnosis. The presence and nature of any focal onset or aura is of the greatest significance, as it suggests and may localise an epileptic focus. Clinical examination in the idiopathic epilepsies is usually normal outside the ictal and postictal phases, apart from any side effects of drugs. Focal epilepsy may indicate focal brain disease; of patients with focal epilepsy presenting after the age of 30, some 20% have an identifiable cerebral lesion. True petit mal epilepsy is always primary rather than symptomatic, and usually the attacks appear in childhood and disappear in adolescence or early adulthood.

Table 4.1. Drug treatment of different seizure types (International classification)

Seizure type	Drugs of choice
Generalised epilepsies	
1. Absences	
A. Typical	Valproate
B. Atypical	Ethosuximide
2. Epileptic myoclonus	
A. Adolescent	Valproate
B. Childhood	Clonazepam
	Phenytoin
3. Tonic–clonic	Carbamazepine
	Primidone
	Phenobarbitone
	Valproate
4. Tonic seizures	Phenytoin
	Carbamazepine
5. Atonic seizures	Valproate
	Clonazepam
Partial epilepsies	
1. Simple partial (rolandic)	Carbamazepine
2. Complex partial	Phenytoin
A. Simple focal onset	Primidone
B. Impaired consciousness at onset	Phenobarbitone
Secondary generalised epilepsies	
1. Simple or complex partial, evolving to tonic–clonic	Phenytoin
	Carbamazepine
2. Infantile spasms	ACTH
	Clonazepam
3. Myoclonic astatic/atonic (Lennox–Gastaut)	Valproate
	Clonazepam
4. Progressive myoclonic epilepsies with dementia	Carbamazepine
	Phenytoin
Unclassified seizures	

Advice

Patients are advised as far as possible to lead a normal life. Normal education, physical pursuits and occupations are followed unless there is some accompanying disability such as mental handicap. However, working at heights, working with dangerous machinery and driving are incompatible with a continuing liability to attacks.

Driving

1. Recurrent attacks result in a driving ban for 2 years in the United Kingdom, unless they are exclusively nocturnal. After this time the licence can be regained even if the patient is taking anticonvulsant drugs, as long as

there are no attacks during wakefulness. If attacks recur after this time when drugs are reduced or withdrawn on the doctor's advice, then when treatment is restored the driving ban need be reintroduced for only 6 months.

2. After a single fit, patients are instructed not to drive for 6 months, during which time appropriate investigations are done. If these do not reveal a lesion liable to cause recurrent attacks, and no further attacks occur, driving can be reinstated.

3. Driving as a profession is advised against if any fits in adult life have occurred; and the regulations for pilot, heavy goods vehicle and public service vehicle licences are more rigorous still, requiring no fits after the age of 3 years.

Provocation of Fits

Some patients' fits are precipitated by circumstances. In many cases major seizures occur only or mainly after alcohol consumption, loss of sleep, fatigue or at times of stress. Patients are advised to avoid these provocations, in particular alcohol and sleep deprivation, but such advice is not normally considered to be a substitute for drug treatment.

Some (presumably focal) attacks are precipitated by very specific stimuli. The commonest example nowadays is probably the precipitation of fits in photosensitive patients by a flickering television, or by stroboscopic lamps. There are many rarer forms of evoked epilepsy (reading, music, sudden noise or sudden movement are examples of stimuli), many of which occur in circumstances that are harder to avoid than a flickering television. Although binocular stimulation is more hazardous than monocular in photic sensitivity, even approaching a flickering television with a hand over one eye is not entirely safe.

Drug Treatment

When Should Drug Treatment of Fits be Started?

Patients with recurrent epileptic seizures should always be treated with an anticonvulsant drug, whether or not their seizures are secondary to identifiable cerebral or other disease. Treatable underlying causes, such as meningioma, hepatic encephalopathy or uraemia, are dealt with in their own right, as well as the fits.

A difficulty arises when deciding whether to start treatment in subjects who have had their first fit. How likely is it that further seizures will occur? Many people present with a single fit, and often no underlying cause is found on investigation. The proportion who, if untreated, will have another fit within 3 years varies with the population being considered, but is probably not less than 30% in young otherwise fit people. If investigation reveals an underlying cause, the probability of further fits is much higher. If the first occurred under circumstances of great provocation (e.g. acute metabolic upset), then the probability may be lower. Clearly, the more seizures a patient has had, the more likely are further attacks. The likelihood of further fits must be weighed against the inconvenience and possible complications of anticonvulsant treatment.

The conventional threshold for instituting long-term drug treatment is after two definite seizures, occurring on separate occasions; but the question whether and how to treat after a single fit is still a matter of active debate. Most neurologists treat after a single fit only if an epileptogenic lesion is revealed by investigation. Whether in fact drug treatment for a limited period after a first fit, as is sometimes practised, can reduce the likelihood of developing chronic epilepsy (perhaps by blocking a kindling mechanism) is unknown.

The question of treatment after a single aura (or focal seizure not becoming generalised, or petit mal attack) is similar, but arises much less often. These types of epilepsy are not usually diagnosed (or even reported to a doctor) after the first attack, as they are so much less alarming than a grand mal seizure.

Drug Level Monitoring

The aim of drug treatment in epilepsy is to achieve and maintain a dosage of an appropriate drug (see Table 4.1) adequate to prevent attacks without undue toxic effects. The therapeutic drug effect is monitored by recording the frequency, type and severity of any fits. If fits occur, the dosage is increased, measurements of plasma level being of most value to avoid entering the range where symptoms of acute toxicity are likely.

Measuring plasma anticonvulsant drug levels is useful:

1. When using drugs where absorption or metabolic capacity are variable or unpredictable
2. Where there is a low therapeutic ratio
3. Where toxicity can be hard to recognise clinically
4. Where overdosage can lead to fits
5. As a check on compliance

Monitoring plasma drug concentrations is not likely to be very useful where half-life is short, where the therapeutic effect does not closely match the plasma concentration or where receptor tolerance develops. These problems are discussed under the individual drugs.

The upper limit of the therapeutic range (Table 4.2) is the level above which symptoms of acute toxicity (Table 4.3) become common, although in

Table 4.2. Dosages of principal anticonvulsants; (a) = adults, (c) = children

Drug	Starting daily dose (mg)	Mean daily dose (mg/kg)	Time to steady state (days)	Therapeutic range (mg/l)	Serum half-life (h)	Protein binding (%)
Valproate	50–100 (c) 250 (a)	25 (c) 20 (a)	2–4	50–100	4–14 (c) 7–17 (a)	90–95
Ethosuximide	250	15–40 (c) 15–30 (a)	6 (c) 12 (a)	40–100 50–60 (a)	30 (c) 30–60 (a)	0
Carbamazepine	100–200	15–20 (c) 10–20 (a)	3–6	4–12	40–50 (naive) 15–16 (c) 10–18 (a)	67–81
Phenytoin	200 (standard; 900 (loading)	5–15 (c) 5 (a)	5–10	10–20	4–11 (c) 22–40 (a)	65 (infant) 88–92 (a,c)
Primidone	50–125	10	1–5	4–12	16	0–20
Phenobarbitone	30–60	2–4	16–21	10–35	50 (c) 50–96 (a)	50

Table 4.3. Side effects of anticonvulsants

Drug	Dose-related	Idiosyncratic	Long-term	Pregnancy	Monitoring
Ethosuximide	GI upset Ataxia Sedation	Precipitate grand mal Anaemia, leucopenia Abnormal LFTs		Not known	FBC (regularly) LFTs (occasionally)
Na valproate	Sedation Nausea Vomiting	Hepatotoxicity[a] Haemorrhage Transient hair loss		Teratogenic in animals	LFTs (early) FBC
Phenytoin	GI upset Ataxia Nystagmus	Rash Leucopenia SLE-like syndrome	Osteomalacia Megaloblastic anaemia Hirsutism, acne Gum hypertrophy	Teratogenic	FBC (regularly) Drug level Vitamin B_{12}, folate if macrocytic
Carbamazepine	Giddiness Diplopia GI upset	Rash Jaundice Aplastic anaemia		Probably teratogenic	FBC (frequently, initially) LFTs
Phenobarbitone	Sedation Ataxia	Rash Irritability[b]	Megaloblastic anaemia Osteomalacia	Not known	FBC Ca^{2+} Vitamin B_{12}, folate if macrocytic
Primidone	Sedation Dizziness Ataxia	Rash Irritability[b]	Megaloblastic anaemia	Not known	FBC, Ca^{2+} Vitamin B_{12}, folate if macrocytic
Clonazepam	Sedation		Dependence	Not known	
Diazepam	Sedation		Dependence	Not known	

[a] 1/50 000 approximately, usually occurring in the first 6 months
[b] Mainly in children

isolated cases it may need to be exceeded. Chronic and idiosyncratic side effects of anticonvulsant drugs (which will be discussed later) can occur regardless of excellent control of the plasma level.

The lower limit of the therapeutic range (Table 4.2) is probably not real, since many patients can be kept fit-free far below these limits. This may be particularly noticeable when treatment is being slowly and unsuccessfully withdrawn; a patient who remains fit-free on a very low plasma level may then have recurrent fits when the drug is finally stopped.

Metabolism of Anticonvulsants

Most anticonvulsant drugs are in part metabolised by hepatic microsomal enzymes, whose activity is increased ("induced") by some anticonvulsants and some other drugs. Anticonvulsant drugs in previously untreated patients are therefore started at a modest dose and increased thereafter, both so as to gauge the level at which the drug becomes effective and so as not to reach toxic levels in the naive patient. A second drug may further induce microsomal enzymes metabolising a first, leading to a fall in the plasma level of the first drug. Alternatively, different drugs may compete for binding to microsomal enzymes, so a second drug may inhibit the metabolism of the first, and push it into the toxic range. Drugs may compete for binding to plasma proteins. In this case, adding a second drug may precipitate toxicity from the first by increasing the unbound, active, drug level. Drug interactions of these sorts are discussed under the headings of the individual drugs.

Drug Kinetics

With many anticonvulsant drugs used alone the rate of metabolism, and therefore the steady state plasma level, is approximately proportional to the dose (first-order kinetics), but an important exception is phenytoin, which is lipid-soluble and metabolised in the liver, and which saturates the hepatic microsomal system within the therapeutic range (kinetics then approaching zero-order). Thereafter, a small increase in dosage will result in increased half-life and hence a much larger than proportionate rise in plasma level. When hepatic metabolism is saturated, more phenytoin is excreted unchanged in the urine. The dosage of phenytoin required to give a therapeutic plasma level may vary widely between different individuals, according to hepatic enzyme capacity. The relationship between dose and plasma level is somewhat more predictable if dose is standardised on body surface area, rather than body weight, but even this is not reliable enough to be a substitute for measurement of plasma or salivary levels (see Table 4.2).

The initial choice of drug in different forms of epilepsy is given in Table 4.1, and pharmacokinetic properties of the first-line anticonvulsant drugs in Table 4.2. In general, petit mal is treated with sodium valproate, ethosuximide or clonazepam. For nonfocal idiopathic grand mal seizures the drugs of choice include sodium valproate or phenytoin. Partial epilepsies, including grand mal seizures with a focal aura, are treated with one or more of four drugs (phenytoin, carbamazepine, phenobarbitone and primidone). Phenytoin and carbamazepine are considered to be superior to the other drugs in many patients because of their much lesser sedative effect.

First-Line Drugs

Ethosuximide

Ethosuximide is perhaps still the first-line drug for the treatment of petit mal absence attacks, where there are no grand mal seizures and the EEG shows typical 3 per second spike-and-wave activity.

Ethosuximide is rapidly and completely absorbed, and has a long plasma half-life so a steady state is not reached for 6 days in children, 12 in adults. Kinetics are nearly first-order, with an insignificant tendency to enzyme saturation. As ethosuximide is unbound in plasma, salivary levels are close to plasma levels. Metabolites are inactive, and 10%–20% is excreted unchanged.

Ethosuximide can increase liability to tonic–clonic seizures, so if these subsequently start, either another drug such as phenytoin is added, or sodium valproate is substituted for ethosuximide.

Sodium Valproate

This drug (a derivative of 2-propylpentanoic acid) is active in controlling both petit mal absence and tonic–clonic grand mal seizures, so it may be the drug of choice in young people suffering from both forms of epilepsy, which is not uncommon. It is also effective in juvenile myoclonic epilepsy and in grand mal in adults. Attention and alertness is often improved in children transferred from ethosuximide to sodium valproate, so some authorities now prefer sodium valproate to ethosuximide in petit mal.

Sodium valproate (the acid, amide or magnesium salt are used in some countries) causes gastric irritation and nausea. It can be taken in enteric form or after meals, so as to slow absorption, building the dose up slowly, with single doses not exceeding 600 mg (daily dose up to 30 mg/kg for adults). Sodium valproate displaces plasma-bound drugs, and may therefore precipitate toxicity if phenytoin, phenobarbitone or primidone are being given as well. In low concentrations, valproate is mainly bound to plasma proteins, but this binding saturates as the plasma level rises, so the half-life becomes shorter with increasing dose. Salivary levels are of no value, as valproate does not pass into saliva. High dosages can cause a bleeding tendency. Liver failure occasionally (1 in 50 000 patients) occurs, usually in the first 6 months, but not necessarily in high dosage. Liver function tests should therefore be repeated at least during that time, in order to detect any sign of impending liver damage. Less serious but more common side effects of sodium valproate include hair loss and weight gain.

Sodium valproate probably acts by long-term inhibition of enzymes which degrade GABA. The antiepileptic activity of a single dose (mediated by increased levels of brain GABA) therefore may outlast the plasma level. It is water-soluble, so it enters brain slowly and the free-drug level in the brain is low. Valproate is oxidised to inert metabolites, and very little is excreted unchanged.

Phenytoin

Phenytoin is a powerful and effective anticonvulsant, but often causes acute toxic side effects (most often nystagmus and ataxia) at only a little above the optimum therapeutic range. This fact, combined with the microsomal enzyme saturation and zero-order kinetics in the therapeutic range, and high protein binding, means that small, not large, adjustments of phenytoin dosage are necessary for best control. Missing a single or a few doses may cause major alterations in plasma levels.

For many years the pharmacokinetics of phenytoin were not widely appreciated, and adult patients were often treated with a standard dosage of 100 mg three times daily. When the long half-life and the need for fine dose adjustments became known, and plasma level assays became routine, treatment became more effective and the manufacturers introduced a 25-mg capsule. The plasma half-life of phenytoin is sufficiently long that it can often be given once a day, usually in the evening; the half-life lengthens as the plasma level rises and metabolic saturation occurs. The time taken to reach a steady state after the start of treatment may be as long as 2 weeks. It is shorter in children, as the half-life is shorter (see Table 4.2). Phenytoin should therefore be given to children in twice daily divided doses. Adding phenytoin in a patient already on carbamazepine often shortens the plasma half-life of carbamazepine by hepatic enzyme induction.

Acute phenytoin toxicity can be precipitated by giving diazepam (which prolongs the half-life of phenytoin). Acute toxicity can also be precipitated by changing from one formulation of phenytoin to another, as there can be a difference of bioavailability between various preparations. For example, phenytoin sodium is much more soluble than phenytoin base. Phenytoin sodium or finely divided phenytoin base are both absorbed rapidly, but macrocrystalline or amorphous phenytoin base is absorbed only slowly. Phenytoin sodium may precipitate in gastric acid as finely divided phenytoin base.

Even when the plasma level is nearer the lower than higher end of the therapeutic range, any dosage increment of phenytoin should not exceed one-sixth of the dose, in order to avoid precipitating toxicity. Some patients' fits are well controlled at blood levels that are well below the accepted therapeutic range. Salivary phenytoin level is equivalent to the level of free (unbound) phenytoin in plasma, so it is (at least theoretically) more appropriate than plasma level. The fraction bound to albumin varies in normal plasma between 80% and 90%, so the active (unbound) level may differ by as much as a factor of two, for a given total plasma level. However, phenytoin binds to brain about as well as it does to albumin, so the theoretical advantage of salivary over plasma levels may not be real. This depends on the kinetics of brain binding, and whether the anticonvulsant effect is exerted by bound or unbound brain phenytoin.

Chronic Toxicity

Besides the acute effects of overdosage, phenytoin causes many chronic toxic effects (see Table 4.3). These may occur despite good control of plasma level within the optimum therapeutic range. Long-term treatment can cause gum hypertrophy, coarsening of facial features, acne, increased body hair, a macrocytic anaemia probably due to a functional folate deficiency, and vitamin D deficiency resulting in osteomalacia.

Phenytoin increases the rate of metabolism of many drugs, including anticoagulants and steroids, and should not be given in conjunction with the low-dose contraceptive pill (which may be rendered ineffective). In women of childbearing age, carbamazepine or sodium valproate are now more commonly used than phenytoin. Teratogenic effects of anticonvulsants including phenytoin are discussed in the section on epilepsy and pregnancy.

Carbamazepine

Carbamazepine is an increasingly used anticonvulsant as it does not cause hirsutism, acne, gum hypertrophy, or coarsening of the features. However, giddiness and diplopia due to a toxic blood level are common, particularly if a full dose is given at first, and the preferred method is for the full dosage to be introduced slowly (while hepatic enzyme induction occurs). Hepatic microsomal enzyme autoinduction (resulting in a fall in plasma carbamazepine level) occurs both with time and with increasing dosage, so that an increase in dose results in a less than proportionate rise in plasma level. This autoinduction is variable, and carbamazepine absorption is incomplete, so plasma levels cannot be accurately predicted from the dose. Individual doses should not exceed 400 mg, because of the likelihood of nausea and increasingly incomplete absorption. Carbamazepine increases the rate of metabolism of phenytoin. The 10,11-epoxide metabolite has some anticonvulsant activity, and is about 50% bound to albumin. Very little carbamazepine is excreted unchanged. Carbamazepine is lipid-soluble and penetrates brain well.

Carbamazepine (in contrast with barbiturates) causes much less impairment of mood and cognitive ability in children with chronic epilepsy, and reduction in fit frequency may result in an actual improvement in behaviour and learning. Some authorities believe that carbamazepine has a positive psychotropic effect in adults and children.

Idiosyncratic early side effects such as jaundice, rash, oedema and anaemia indicating drug sensitivity are relatively common with carbamazepine. These necessitate change to another drug. Aplastic anaemia and hepatic failure occur very rarely, and in practice only in patients whose drug sensitivity has been signalled by a skin rash, but ignored. Routine repeated blood counts and liver function tests in people taking carbamazepine are therefore probably not justified. The plasma half-life of carbamazepine is long in the naive patient, but because of autoinduction when given regularly the half-life becomes relatively short (so the drug must be given at least twice a day), and is further shortened by other drugs which cause further enzyme induction (see Table 4.2). Protein binding is not affected by the presence of other drugs. Salivary level is equivalent to free (unbound) plasma level.

Phenobarbitone

Phenobarbitone, introduced in 1912, was the first really effective anticonvulsant, more powerful and with less side effects than the bromides introduced by Queen Victoria's accoucheur, Sir Charles Locock, in the 1850s. Phenobarbitone is still sometimes used to prevent infantile febrile convulsions, and many adults with grand mal or occasional focal seizures who have been on phenobarbitone for many years remain well controlled. Phenobarbitone is cheap and simple to administer.

Phenobarbitone is absorbed completely, but at a rather variable rate. It is loosely bound to plasma protein, and binding is increased by acidosis. Phenobarbitone intoxication is therefore treated by alkaline diuresis, which unbinds phenobarbitone and greatly increases the rate of renal excretion. It is eliminated by first-order kinetics, so that the plasma level is proportional to dose over the therapeutic range. The half-life is shorter in children (see Table 4.2). Salivary phenobarbitone levels are unreliable, being pH-dependent. The metabolism of phenobarbitone is often slowed by competition with phenytoin when this is given concurrently.

Phenobarbitone can exacerbate or precipitate petit mal in children. Drowsiness and loss of concentration are its most prominent side effects, particularly when treatment is first started, so phenobarbitone is not a drug of first choice in either adults or children. Unlike phenytoin and most other anticonvulsants, it is saleable as an illicit drug and can cause dependence, and it can cause fatal respiratory depression in overdosage. Sudden withdrawal is liable to provoke withdrawal fits which are resistant except to reintroducing the drug; so withdrawal of phenobarbitone is always done slowly.

Primidone

Primidone is an anticonvulsant in its own right, but part of its anticonvulsant effect is due to phenobarbitone metabolically derived from it. The rate at which primidone is metabolised to phenobarbitone and phenylethylmalona-mide varies widely between individuals, and phenobarbitone formation is increased by concurrent treatment with other anticonvulsants (e.g. phenytoin or carbamazepine). In children, up to two-thirds of a dose of primidone may be excreted unchanged. Although most anticonvulsants have some sedative effect, this is very marked with primidone, as with phenobarbitone. On starting treatment with primidone, dizziness and sedation are often particularly prominent, so it is started at about one-quarter the maintenance dosage, increasing over 2–3 weeks to 250 mg twice daily, after which the dose is controlled by clinical response and plasma level. Since primidone is almost unbound, the salivary level is similar to the plasma level.

Adjunctive Drugs

Benzodiazepines

Diazepam, clobazam and clonazepam are often used as adjuncts to the major drugs in the control of epilepsy, whether grand mal, focal or petit mal with 3 per second spike-and-wave. Their antiepileptic activity if used alone is good at first, but not always sustained. Intravenous or rectal benzodiazepines, usually diazepam, are an essential part of the treatment of status epilepticus (to be discussed later). Diazepam is very poorly absorbed intramuscularly, so this route is not used. It is rapidly absorbed orally, with a half-life of 20–60 h. An active metabolite (n-desmethyldiazepam) is formed which has an even longer half-life (30–90 h). Diazepam infused into the rectum is well absorbed, but suppositories have been found to absorb poorly (this is found to depend on the type of capsulation). It is 97% bound to plasma proteins, and the free 3% equilibrates with CSF and saliva. Very little diazepam is excreted unchanged. The indications for clobazam are similar to those for diazepam. Initial dosage is 20–30 mg/day for adults, increasing if necessary to 60 mg/day in divided doses.

Clonazepam

Clonazepam (0.1 mg kg^{-1} day^{-1}) is rapidly absorbed, 85% bound to plasma proteins, and metabolised to inactive products with an elimination half-life of 20–60 h (adults) or 20–30 h (children). Enzyme induction by other anticonvulsants can shorten the half-life and lower the level. Clonazepam is used in focal, nonfocal and particularly myoclonic epilepsy.

Sulthiame

Sulthiame is absorbed rapidly and excreted mainly unchanged in the urine. Its antiepileptic activity is derived largely from its inhibition of the metabolism of phenytoin given concurrently, so increasing the phenytoin plasma level. The only rational indication for sulthiame therefore is to enable phenytoin to be given once daily to patients where this is required, and whose phenytoin half-life is otherwise too short.

Other Drugs

Other anticonvulsants used in the past, mostly closely related structurally to one or other of the first-line drugs, are now considered to carry disadvantages with no compensating advantage, when compared with their first-line stablemates.

Treatment Problems

Status Epilepticus

Status is present when fits recur without full recovery of consciousness between them. Grand mal status is life-threatening (mortality 20%–50% untreated, up to 10% treated) and is a medical emergency. It can cause brain damage, particularly in children. Focal motor status (epilepsia partialis continua) and petit mal status do not carry the same danger to life, but complex partial status can cause permanent memory deficit. For many years paraldehyde 10 ml i.m. from a glass syringe, or 0.05–0.1 ml/kg infused in normal saline was the standard (and effective) treatment, but sterile abscess at an injection site and thrombophlebitis at an infusion site were common sequelae.

A number of different (alternative) regimes for the initial management of status have been advocated in recent years, using diazepam, clonazepam, chlormethiazole or phenytoin. There appears to be little to choose between them in the initial management of status; what matters is that the operator is familiar with one technique, and enough drug is given to stop the fits, but not to depress respiration severely. Some methods in current use are as follows:

1. Diazepam may be given i.v. in a bolus of 10 mg every 15 min until the fits are controlled or until 50–60 mg has been given. Alternatively, diazepam can be given by infusion at 2 mg/min; in 80% of cases, the fits cease within 10 min.

2. Chlormethiazole (which is rapidly metabolised) infused at 0.7 g/h or

3. Clonazepam (up to 0.1 mg/kg i.v.) are effective alternatives, and many succeed where diazepam has failed. Benzodiazepines are also particularly

effective in petit mal (absence) status and in children. They are poorly soluble in infusion solutions, so when infusion is required diazepam 20 mg injection should be diluted with 250 ml 5% or 10% glucose, a sufficient volume to prevent microprecipitation. Benzodiazepines are never given i.m., as they are absorbed far too slowly to be useful. Injections or infusions of diazepam should be given into a large vein as there is a tendency to cause thrombophlebitis; the vehicle in which it is solubilised is irritant. Diazepam is short-acting and it is essential to introduce a long-acting drug such as phenytoin at the same time, so as to prevent recurrence of the status.

4. If phenytoin is to be used, it is essential first to ascertain whether the patient is already taking it. If not, then parenteral phenytoin can be given by slow intravenous injection of up to 250 mg. The rate of injection should not exceed 50 mg/min, and the ECG should be monitored (beware heart block). If seizures continue 30 min after the start of the injection, a further slow i.v. injection up to a total of 400 mg can be given. Oral or intramuscular phenytoin to complete a loading dose of 15 mg/kg (900 mg for a 60-kg adult) can then be given. Parenteral phenytoin is alkaline and cannot be added to intravenous infusions, as it will precipitate. For patients believed to be already on phenytoin, blood is first taken for a phenytoin level, and then the slow i.v. injection is given, but not the remainder of the loading dose. Subsequent dosage is adjusted according to the serum phenytoin level.

For serial untreated epilepsy (but not major status epilepticus), a loading dose of phenytoin can be given orally over a few hours (300 mg 3-hourly, so as to avoid vomiting). This is likely to achieve a therapeutic blood level in not less than 24 h. In either case, after initial phenytoin loading, and if phenytoin is to be continued, it can be given (after the first day) at 300 mg/day, plasma concentration measured after 1 week, and then phenytoin dose adjusted accordingly.

In major status epilepticus, the combination of a full intravenous loading dose of phenytoin together with an infusion of diazepam or chlormethiazole usually stops the fits within an hour. If it does not, then the patient should be transferred to an intensive care unit and treated with thiopentone and a muscular relaxant while the anticonvulsants work. This necessitates intubation and positive pressure respiration; and although the convulsion is abolished, the neural discharges are not; brain damage may not be prevented by this means. Anticonvulsants must therefore be continued throughout.

Infusion of phenobarbitone (5 mg/kg) or paraldehyde (4%) or lignocaine (50–100 mg) may succeed where the first-line methods fail, but a combination of diazepam and phenobarbitone may cause respiratory failure, and should therefore be avoided. These drugs therefore add unnecessary complication and risk, and we do not recommend their routine use.

In all cases of status, it is necessary to secure the airway, set up a drip in a large vein, take venous blood for glucose, urea, electrolytes and drug levels, and if necessary arterial blood for gases. Glucose solution 10% and vitamin B complex can be infused initially, and later infusions are calculated to correct electrolyte abnormalities. Tepid sponging and correction of acidosis may be needed.

Epilepsy and Pregnancy (see Table 4.3)

Untreated maternal seizures are considered a greater risk to the foetus than well-controlled anticonvulsant medication, which is therefore not withdrawn when pregnancies are planned, unless the risk of further fits is thought to be very low. There is a well-documented increase (roughly a doubling) in the incidence of foetal malformation in babies exposed to phenytoin in utero (often distressing craniofacial defects such as harelip, microcephaly and mental retardation). Carbamazepine has also recently been associated with retardation of foetal head growth, and sodium valproate with spina bifida. It is not certain that these effects are entirely due to the antifolate action of many anticonvulsants, but folic acid supplementation in women on anticonvulsants and who are pregnant or likely to become pregnant is considered necessary. This is unlikely to result in recurrent fits, and is preferable to withdrawing or changing anticonvulsants. Anticonvulsant requirements increase during pregnancy and fall after delivery, so plasma levels need to be checked more frequently and dosages adjusted accordingly. The requirement during pregnancy is increased by greater maternal hepatic enzyme activity, and later to a small extent by the addition of the foetal liver. Postpartum drug requirement usually falls rapidly to the nonpregnant state, so toxicity can easily occur at that time. Secretion of anticonvulsants into breast milk is negligible except in the case of ethosuximide, and even then it is seldom significant (i.e. it does not reach toxic levels), even though the neonatal liver metabolises drugs slowly.

Febrile Fits and Other Fits in Children

Fits in children may occur in relation to acute febrile illnesses or biochemical disturbances, which should be treated appropriately by antibiotics or electrolyte correction, and by tepid sponging. Febrile convulsions, if prolonged or repeated, may lead to later chronic epilepsy, particularly psychomotor epilepsy, in association with mesial temporal sclerosis; the hippocampus is particularly sensitive to ischaemic damage during fits, and when scarred it often subsequently becomes epileptogenic. Febrile convulsions may be treated with i.v. diazepam (up to 1 mg/kg), followed by prophylaxis with phenobarbitone. It is conventional to treat with phenobarbitone ($3\text{--}4$ mg kg^{-1} day^{-1}) continuously, supplemented by 30 mg per year of age at the onset of any subsequent fever. An alternative is to give rectal soft gelatine (rapidly absorbed) formulation diazepam suppositories with the onset of fever.

For major and minor fits not associated with fever in children, sodium valproate is often satisfactory. Attention and alertness may improve when other drugs (such as ethosuximide) are withdrawn. Infantile spasms may follow immunisation (e.g. pertussis) or may be cause by disorders such as tuberose sclerosis or cerebral lipidoses. In the latter cases, the spasms are difficult to control, and are associated with mental handicap. ACTH 20–30 units/day for 3–4 weeks is regarded as the treatment of choice, accompanied and followed by benzodiazepines.

Genetic Counselling

Two questions often arise. The first and most common is asked by people with idiopathic or acquired epilepsy who are contemplating starting a family: what is the chance of a child of theirs developing epilepsy? The second comes from normal parents of an epileptic child, who want to know the probability of further children being affected. Some relevant observations concerning major seizures are:

1. The prevalence of epilepsy in the general population is about 0.75%.

2. If one parent has epilepsy, the incidence in children is about 2%–3%.

3. If both parents have epilepsy, the incidence rises to 25%.

4. If one parent has epilepsy and the other an "unstable" EEG, then the risk may be intermediate.

5. Risk is also increased in the children of people with some types of acquired epilepsy (e.g. post-traumatic or following febrile convulsions).

6. A family history of fits (in first-degree relations) is often found in children with febrile convulsions (50%) or fits generally (30%).

A reasonable interpretation of these observations would be that a postulated tendency to seizures is inherited polygenically, at least some of the genes being recessive. Such a tendency may in some instances never be expressed as fits except under provocation (e.g. fever in infancy; head injury, alcohol or metabolic insult at any age). Some authorities believe this postulated tendency can be detected as EEG instability.

For petit mal the picture is more clear-cut, as about 40% of sibs of children with petit mal also have a spike-and-wave abnormality, suggesting an autosomal dominant inheritance. Certain of the neurological syndromes with associated epilepsy are also inherited as autosomal dominants (e.g. tuberose sclerosis, neurofibromatosis, Huntington's disease), although formes frustes are common in the first two examples.

Other neurological syndromes with epilepsy are inherited as autosomal recessives (e.g. lipidosis, galactosaemia, mucopolysaccharidoses, Unverricht's myoclonic epilepsy, phenylketonuria and maple syrup urine disease). Here, what is usually called for is advice after the birth of an affected child, concerning the risk to further children, which is likely to be about 25%.

Clinical rarities that may have been described in several generations of a single family usually have an autosomal dominant inheritance. On the other hand, a family history is relatively rare in children with isolated infantile spasms (5%) or Lennox–Gastaut syndrome (7%).

Anticonvulsants and Liver Disease

Hepatocellular disease will both slow metabolism and be associated with hypoalbuminaemia. Hypoalbuminaemia may lead to toxicity at "normal" total plasma levels (remembering that it is the unbound fraction that is active). Salivary levels may be more appropriate in such patients, at least for those drugs (q.v.) where salivary levels are reliable. Portosystemic shunting in liver disease (either via varices or a surgical shunt) may increase drug bioavailability by reducing first-pass metabolism. For all these reasons, the right dose will be smaller and given at longer intervals.

Anticonvulsants and Renal Disease

Plasma protein binding may be reduced in renal failure, and albumin levels reduced, so that the unbound fraction is increased, and the upper therapeutic range therefore reduced. The half-life of drugs excreted by the kidney (e.g. phenobarbitone) is prolonged.

One Drug or More?

In the past polypharmacy was usual, patients being started on two or more drugs simultaneously as a routine, in standard dosage. This is now seen as irrational, since as many as 80% of patients are fully controlled on one drug, when the dosage is properly tailored to their needs. Mixed types of seizure may be a reason for maintenance on more than one drug, but sodium valproate may often control major seizures and petit mal simultaneously.

Pharmacokinetic interactions between drugs can make for difficulty in the control of plasma levels when more than one drug is in use. Therefore, if a drug of choice is ineffective, a second drug is substituted (rather than added) in a gradual changeover. However, if a drug seems to be partially effective, a second drug can be added, and its dosage adjusted under control of plasma levels. Dosage of the first drug may then need to be adjusted if the second is one that alters its rate of metabolism. In a few instances, if the second drug fails to produce further improvement, it may be withdrawn and yet another drug introduced. Since different anticonvulsants are believed to act at different neuronal sites and by different mechanisms, it is not irrational to expect that combination therapy will occasionally be superior to monotherapy, but this is usually outweighed by the extra complication of drug interactions and the increased likelihood of noncompliance.

Do Patients Take Their Tablets?

It has been estimated that only about 50% of all tablets are taken as directed, and anticonvulsants are not likely to be an exception. They are taken long-term, sometimes in complex schedules; they can impair concentration and memory, can cause other toxic effects, and may need to be taken several times a day, all factors which reduce compliance.

Compliance is likely to be improved therefore by eliminating polypharmacy, by a once- or twice-daily schedule (as part of the morning and bedtime routines) where possible, or by asking the patient to carry the day's tablets in a small box as an aide-mémoire. Monitoring of plasma levels checks compliance and minimises the chance of acute toxicity. If levels are persistently low and fits uncontrolled, admitting the patient for treatment under supervision may solve the problem.

Surgery

Temporal Lobectomy

When complex partial seizures (psychomotor attacks) are not well controlled, a change of drug, dosage or combination may sometimes be successful, or a reduction in stress, alcohol or fit-precipitating stimuli. If fits remain severe in spite of the best medical treatment, then temporal lobectomy may be considered if the patient is otherwise suitable. This requires careful and specialist assessment in an epilepsy unit to determine the exact site of the focus and whether or not it can be removed without damaging memory or speech. Multiple bilateral neurological signs, multiple epileptic foci on EEG, psychosis or mental handicap normally contraindicate surgical treatment of epilepsy. In appropriately selected cases the results of temporal lobectomy are good or excellent in 60%–80% of patients. Other surgery for epilepsy (e.g. hemispherectomy) is still occasionally done, but again is confined to specialist centres.

Follow-up

Long-term follow-up in epilepsy is necessary for:

1. Adjusting dosage
2. Detecting chronic toxic effects
3. Advising on driving, occupation, pregnancy, travel, genetic counselling (all problems which can arise after satisfactory control has been achieved)
4. Withdrawing treatment at appropriate time

The first three of these aims have already been dealt with.

When to Withdraw Treatment

A majority (perhaps 80%) of all patients started on anticonvulsant treatment after two or more fits will cease to have fits on treatment. How long should this be continued? Anticonvulsants are toxic, but however long a patient has been fit-free on anticonvulsants, there is always a chance that attacks may recur when treatment is withdrawn. The decision is therefore a balanced judgement. Gradual withdrawal after 3 fit-free years is a useful guide in adults with nonfocal seizures. Patients with focal fits should continue on treatment indefinitely if they have even slight "auras" on treatment.

Patients with only a few (2–4) grand mal seizures prior to treatment, and who are completely fit-free on anticonvulsant drug treatment (for 2 or more years) have a 50%–60% chance of remaining fit-free for at least 2 years after withdrawal. The occurrence of a large number of grand mal fits or of focal fits, or the occurrence of more than one type of fit, or the presence of an identifiable structural cause, are all factors associated both with a poor response to drugs and with an increased rate of recurrence on withdrawal. If there are abnormal neurological signs, mental handicap or psychosis, fits are likely to be more difficult to control, and are likely to recur if treatment is stopped. Also, if the EEG during treatment remains grossly abnormal despite freedom from attacks, drug withdrawal may be unsuccessful.

In addition to these factors, the presence or absence of chronic drug toxicity and the age and occupation of the patient should be considered. Early adulthood (25–30 years) is considered a good time for withdrawal in the childhood and adolescent epilepsies, when successful drug withdrawal after several fit-free years on treatment can often be achieved; there is an impression that many children "grow out" of their fits. In one series, children who had been fit-free on treatment for 4 years were found to have a recurrence rate of about 30% after withdrawal, about two-thirds of these recurrences occurring in the first 2 years. Some authorities are of the view that anticonvulsants should not generally be withdrawn in adolescents with a history of childhood fits, as recurrence is both more likely and more upsetting then. Withdrawal should either be achieved in childhood, or else left until early adult life.

If fits recur during gradual drug withdrawal, it is our practice to abandon ideas of drug withdrawal indefinitely, unless there are strong reasons such as chronic toxicity; it may be possible to reduce the dose. If they recur after gradual drug withdrawal has been completed, then restarting a small dose may be enough.

Withdrawal in Petit Mal

The EEG may be helpful in determining whether petit mal has been outgrown. This occurs in about 80% of cases with classic petit mal. Nearly half these patients however have associated grand mal, which remits in only about one-third of cases. Atypical minor attacks remit more rarely, and there is little prospect of drug withdrawal in children with severe epileptic encephalopathy.

Further Reading

Delgado-Escueta AV, Treiman DM, Walsh GO (1983) The treatable epilepsies. N Engl J Med 308: 1508–1514, 1576–1584

Laidlaw J, Richens A (eds) (1980) A textbook of epilepsy. Churchill Livingstone, Edinburgh London Melbourne New York

Pedley TA, Meldrum BS (eds) (1983) Recent advances in epilepsy, vol 1. Churchill Livingstone, London

Pond DA, Espir M (1976) Epilepsy. In:Raffle A (ed) Medical aspects of fitness to drive. Medical Commission on Accident Prevention, London, pp 16–22

5 Treatment of Movement Disorders

Movement disorders comprise a large group of neurological conditions characterised by either: (a) slowness and poverty of movement with rigidity, and sometimes rest tremor—the akinetic–rigid syndrome; or (b) abnormal involuntary movements—the dyskinesias. Common causes of these disorders are shown in Tables 5.1 and 5.2.

Table 5.1. Common causes of the akinetic–rigid syndrome

Disease	Distinguishing features
Parkinson's disease	Lewy bodies
Postencephalitic parkinsonism	Encephalitis lethargica
Drug-induced parkinsonism	Neuroleptic drugs
Progressive supranuclear palsy	Supranuclear gaze palsy
Multiple system atrophies	
Strionigral degeneration	
Olivopontocerebellar degeneration	Cerebellar ataxia and atrophy
Progressive autonomic failure	Autonomic neuropathy
Wilson's disease	Abnormal copper metabolism
Cerebrovascular pseudoparkinsonism	Strokes, lacunae, infarcts
Parkinsonism in hydrocephalus	
In Alzheimer's disease	Dementia
In dementia pugilistica	Boxers

This is not the place to discuss the differential diagnosis of the many conditions that present with movement disorders. Nor will the details of treatment of each of these diseases be considered. In general, treatment of all akinetic–rigid syndromes follows the principles of management of Parkinson's disease. Antiparkinsonian drugs fall into two main classes, the dopamine agonists and the anticholinergics. Treatment of chorea is based on the use of dopamine antagonists, and that of dystonia on anticholinergics. Accordingly, detailed information on drugs acting on brain acetylcholine and dopamine systems is given in the following sections.

Table 5.2. Common causes of dyskinesias

Type of dyskinesia	Disease	Distinguishing features
Tremor	Parkinson's disease	Rest tremor
	Essential (familial) tremor	Postural tremor
	Cerebellar disease	Intention tremor
Chorea	Huntington's disease	Dominant inheritance
	Sydenham's chorea	Streptococcal infection
	Thyrotoxic chorea	
	Lupus chorea	
	Polycythaemic chorea	
	Drug-induced chorea	Neuroleptics, contraceptive pill
Tics	Gilles de la Tourette disease	Vocalisations
Myoclonus	Epileptic myoclonus	Seizures
	Progressive myoclonus epilepsy	
	Storage disease	Dementia
	Cerebellar degeneration	Ataxia
	Metabolic myoclonus	
	Renal, hepatic, respiratory failure	
	Electrolyte imbalance	
	Toxic myoclonus	
	Drugs and poisons	
	Essential (hereditary myoclonus)	
Dystonia	Primary (familial) torsion dystonia	
	Symptomatic dystonia	
	Athetosis	Cerebral palsy
	Wilson's disease	Abnormal copper metabolism
	Lesch–Nyhan disease	Uric acid
	Hallervorden–Spatz disease	Iron
	Drug-induced dystonia	Neuroleptics
	Paroxysmal dystonia	Attacks

Acetylcholine

Acetylcholine is widely distributed in all parts of the nervous system.
Cholinergic projections to all parts of the cerebral cortex arise in the
diencephalic substantia innominata (nucleus basalis of Meynert) and septal
nuclei (nucleus of the diagonal band of Broca). The neostriatum (caudate
nucleus and putamen) contain many cholinergic interneurones, as does the brain
stem reticular formation. In the spinal cord, acetylcholine is the transmitter from
motoneurones to Renshaw cells. Acetylcholine is considered briefly in Chap. 9,
where the role of peripheral muscarinic cholinergic receptors on the muscle
end-plate is considered in relation to myasthenia gravis.

The central nervous system contains both muscarinic and nicotinic
cholinergic receptors, but the relative roles of action of acetylcholine on these
two sites has not been established. Drugs affecting central acetylcholine

systems must be capable of crossing the blood–brain barrier to affect CNS cholinergic targets (see Chap. 9).

Drugs Affecting Central Cholinergic Mechanisms

Receptor Agonists

Nicotine exerts pharmacological actions on the CNS, but is of no therapeutic value. Arecoline is present in betel nuts, chewed in many parts of Asia for a central stimulant effect, as well as for its capacity to increase salivation and improve digestion. Loss of cholinergic innervation to the cerebral cortex, with relative preservation of cortical cholinergic receptors is one of the main biochemical findings in Alzheimer's disease. This has led to attempts to treat the dementia of this disorder by drugs aimed at increasing brain cholinergic activity. Choline (the precursor of acetylcholine), lecithin (a potent source of choline), and deanol (which may act as a precursor of choline), have been tried without benefit. Synthetic acetylcholine agonists are under study, but so far have not achieved success. Physostigmine inhibits CNS acetylcholine esterase, and can briefly improve memory functions, but is not of therapeutic value in this condition.

Receptor Antagonists

Many drugs block the action of acetylcholine, mostly by competitive antagonism. They have mainly atropine-like structures, and occur naturally in deadly nightshade (*Atropa belladonna*), henbane (*Hyoscyamus niger*) and thornapple (*Datura stramonium*). The main alkaloids are hyoscine and hyoscyamine. (Atropine is D,L-hyoscyamine; scopolamine is L-hyoscine.) In addition to the naturally occurring alkaloids, a number of synthetic anticholinergic drugs have been developed, which differ in their duration of action and sedative or stimulant effects.

Muscarinic receptor antagonists (Table 5.3) relax the ciliary muscle and iris circular muscle, cause paralysis of near focus and dilatation of the pupil, raise the intraocular pressure, and may precipitate coma, increase heart rate, reduce airway resistance, and salivary, bronchial, lachrymal and gastrointestinal secretion, block vagally mediated gastric release, reduce gastrointestinal tone and peristalsis and cause urinary retention.

Atropine

L-Hyoscyamine is 20 times more active than the D-isomer. Atropine is completely absorbed after oral administration with a $t_{1/2}$ of 13–38 h. Atropine undergoes hepatic first-pass metabolism and is mostly *N*-methylated and glucuronidated. Between a third and a half of an orally administered dose appears unchanged in the urine. Atropine is a competitive antagonist of the muscarinic effects of acetylcholine, but has little or no neuromuscular blocking activity.

Table 5.3. Synthetic anticholinergic drugs

Drug	Dose	Notes
Atropine methonitrate	200–600 μg p.o.	Agitation, excitement
Atropine sulphate	250–500 μg p.o.	
Hyoscine butylbromide	200 mg i.m.	Sedation
Propantheline bromide	15–45 mg daily	Mainly gastrointestinal action
Emepronium bromide	200–600 mg daily	No central action
Procyclidine hydrochloride	7.5–60 mg daily	Sedative
Benztropine mesylate	1–4 mg p.o. daily	Sedative and cumulative
	(1–2 mg i.m. or i.v.)	(i.v. for acute dystonia)
Benzhexol hydrochloride	5–15 mg p.o. daily	
	(also delayed release)	
Methixine hydrochloride	15–60 mg p.o. daily	
Orphenadrine hydrochloride	150–400 mg p.o. daily	Stimulant
Biperiden	2–6 mg p.o. daily	Sedative

Other compounds with anticholinergic effects: tricyclic drugs; phenothiazines; antihistamines (H-l receptor blocking drugs)

Atropine 0.5 mg s.c. has a powerful effect in reducing secretions and a dual effect on the pulse rate, with initial slowing due to central stimulation followed by acceleration. Scopolamine (hyoscine) is an ester of tropic acid and scopin, and has similar peripheral actions, but depressant central effects, euphoria being followed by drowsiness, amnesia, fatigue and dreamless sleep.

Atropine Substitutes

As well as the natural alkaloids, a number of synthetic anticholinergic drugs have been developed (Table 5.3).

Anticholinergic Toxicity

Centrally acting anticholinergic drugs cause delirium, coma, slow cerebration, inattention, restlessness, aggressive or paranoid behaviour, visual or, less often, tactile hallucinosis, and changes in mood. These side effects may be precipitated by intercurrent infection or simultaneous administration of other drugs with anticholinergic actions. Mental symptoms usually recover within 2–7 days of withdrawal. Chlorpromazine 25–50 mg p.o. will reverse severe restlessness in atropine poisoning. Anticholinergics impair memory in elderly people; 15%–30% of parkinsonian patients develop depression, confusion, delusions or hallucinations on these drugs.

Toxic doses of anticholinergic drugs cause in addition to severe mental changes, widely dilated pupils, flushed dry skin, fever, increased intraocular pressure, tachycardia, palpitations and arrhythmias, urinary retention and constipation, and rapid respiration. Angle-closure glaucoma may be precipitated by anticholinergic drugs, but is very rare. Thymoxamine 0.5% will reverse atropine-induced mydriasis.

Extreme dryness of the mouth may cause gingivitis and tooth loss. Change in diet, addition of roughage, lactulose 5–30 ml daily, ispaghula husk, 3–6 g daily or other laxatives may be required to combat constipation. Neostigmine 1–2 mg s.c. will reverse the peripheral, but not central cholinergic blockade. Eczema, retrosternal pain due to increased oesophageal reflux, and cardiac infarction have all been attributed to anticholinergic drugs.

Dopamine and Noradrenaline (Catecholamines)

A catechol is a benzene ring with two adjacent hydroxyl groups. A catecholamine contains a catechol ring and an amine side chain. Three catecholamines, dopamine, noradrenaline and adrenaline are synthesised in humans. Levodopa, L-dihydroxyphenylalanine, is the precursor amino acid for dopamine, noradrenaline and adrenaline synthesis. The main catecholamines in the CNS are dopamine and noradrenaline.

Localisation of Dopamine and Noradrenaline

The highest concentration of dopamine in the brain is in the basal ganglia. Dopamine neurones in the substantia nigra and adjacent ventral tegmental area give rise to fine axons that project to the neostriatum (caudate nucleus and putamen) and to the nucleus accumbens and other mesolimbic areas. The ventral tegmentum also projects to dopaminergic areas of the cerebral cortex. Other dopaminergic pathways in the brain include those in the hypothalamus concerned with regulation of pituitary function, and a descending system from the diencephalon to the spinal cord.

Noradrenaline neurones lie in the brain stem, mainly in the locus coeruleus and adjacent areas. A dorsal noradrenergic pathway projects to the cerebral cortex; a ventral pathway projects to the hypothalamus. Other pathways project to the cerebellum and spinal cord. The enzymes involved in catecholamine synthesis are shown in Table 5.4.

Dopa Decarboxylase Inhibitors

Two drugs, benserazide (in Madopar) and carbidopa (L-α-methyldopa hydrazine, in Sinemet) are available which inhibit the formation of dopamine

Table 5.4. Enzymes of catecholamine synthesis

Enzyme	Enzyme inhibitor	Clinical use	Effect on blood pressure
Tyrosine hydroxylase[a]	Methyl–p-tyrosine	Phaeochromocytoma	Fall
Aromatic acid (e.g. DOPA) decarboxylase[a,b]	Carbidopa benserazide	Parkinsonism	No change in blood pressure, but potentiates methyldopa, clonidine, hydralazine
	(α-Methyldopa)	Hypertension	Fall
Dopamine β-hydroxylase[c]	Disulfiram diethyldithiocarbonate	Alcoholism	Fall
Monoamine oxidase B	Deprenyl pargyline (low dose)	Prolong action of levodopa	No change
Monoamine oxidase A	Pargyline (high dose)	Depression	Potentiates hypertensive effect of amines
Catechol-O-methyl-transferase	Progesterone		

[a] Requires pteridine (tetrahydropteridine) cofactor, oxygen and ferrous ions as well as niacin.
[b] Pyridoxine dependent. Levodopa peripheral decarboxylation is increased by pyridoxine (vitamin B_6) which prevents the central effect of levodopa given without decarboxylase inhibitor.
[c] Dopamine B hydroxylase contains copper and is inhibited by copper-chelating agents.

from levodopa (as well as the formation of serotonin from 5-hydroxytryptophan, and histamine from histidine). These are both pharmacologically inert and do not prevent endogenous amine synthesis, or by themselves cause hypotension, although they do potentiate the hypotensive action of ganglion-blocking drugs. Both compounds are rapidly absorbed following oral dosage, with peak plasma levels following administration of benserazide 50 mg p.o. at 1 h, and carbidopa 100 mg at 0.5–5 h. Both benserazide and carbidopa are metabolised extensively, with acid metabolites of carbidopa excreted in the urine. No long-term adverse effect has been attributed to either drug.

Since these inhibitors in normal dosage do not enter the brain, the result is to enhance the central, but inhibit the peripheral actions of levodopa. The combination of decarboxylase inhibitors with levodopa in the treatment of parkinsonism has the following advantages:

1. Four- to fivefold reduction in levodopa dosage. Decarboxylase inhibitors cause a four- to fivefold increase in peak plasma levodopa levels, a minor increase of plasma levodopa half-life (of about 10–30 min), and a lower urinary excretion of dopamine and its metabolites.

2. Reduction of emesis from 80% to 15%, owing to the prevention of dopamine formation in the area postrema, which lies outside the blood–brain barrier.

3. Early clinical benefit, in 1–2 weeks rather than 1–2 months.

4. Reduction of cardiac arrhythmias.

5. The addition of pyridoxine does not increase peripheral levodopa metabolism in the presence of inhibitor.

The disadvantages are few and mainly theoretical. Decarboxylase inhibitors may increase the hypotensive effect of ganglion-blocking drugs. Their use combined with levodopa theoretically could cause niacin depletion, but not pellagra in subjects on an adequate diet. Carbidopa will enhance hepatic drug-metabolising enzyme activity, but does not greatly interfere with the action of other drugs that are dependent upon hepatic metabolism. Availability of fixed-ratio levodopa decarboxylase inhibitor tablets, but not the inhibitor alone, sometimes results in too low an intake of inhibitor for total peripheral decarboxylation in subjects on low levodopa dosages.

Dopamine

Dopamine itself is rapidly metabolised, and does not penetrate the brain, so cannot be given orally to replace striatal dopamine deficiency. Dopamine is released into the synaptic cleft from dopamine neurones by exocytosis. This release is calcium-dependent. Many drugs, amphetamine, other phenyl-ethylamines and amantadine, as well as the nerve action potential, cause dopamine release and the drugs may also block neuronal reuptake.

Dopamine receptors are of two main types, D-1 (linked to the enzyme adenylate cyclase), and D-2 (independent of adenylate cyclase). Dopamine and dopamine receptors have a wide distribution at many sites both inside and outside the brain (Table 5.5). Dopamine receptors are also present in mesenteric, renal, coronary and cerebral blood vessels, gastrointestinal tract, autonomic ganglia, ovaries and testes.

Levodopa

Levodopa is pharmacologically inert, but unlike dopamine does cross the blood–brain barrier. The action of levodopa is due mainly to conversion to dopamine and noradrenaline. Although DOPA decarboxylase levels are reduced in the striatum in parkinsonism, presumably sufficient enzyme activity remains to allow for the formation of dopamine from levodopa. Clinical response, dose requirements and tolerance to levodopa vary widely. However, overall, clinical benefit occurs when the plasma concentration of levodopa is high and loss of benefit accompanies falling plasma levels. Clinical response lags approximately 30 min behind plasma levels.

Table 5.5. Dopamine receptor sites

Site	Action of dopamine agonists, [?] e.g. levodopa, ergots	Action of dopamine antagonists, e.g. chlorpromazine, haloperidol
Substantia nigra and striatum	Antiparkinsonian	Cause motor disorders
Hypothalamus	Growth hormone release	Growth hormone inhibition
Pituitary	Prolactin inhibition Growth hormone suppression in acromegaly	Hyperprolactinaemia
Area postrema	Emesis	Antiemetic
Vasomotor centres, blood vessels	Hypotension	Variable effects on blood pressure
Cerebral cortex	Hallucinations	Antipsychotic

Levodopa is of practical value in the treatment of idiopathic Parkinson's disease, postencephalitic parkinsonism and also in drug-induced parkinsonism. High dosages are required owing to rapid extracerebral as well as intracerebral metabolism. Levodopa is the most effective drug available for the treatment of parkinsonism; a great majority of patients improve if the diagnosis is correct.

The usual initial daily oral dosage of levodopa alone is 0.25–1 g in three or more divided doses, or combined with decarboxylase inhibitor, 100–250 mg levodopa three times daily. The dose and time of administration must be established separately in every patient.

Factors Affecting Clinical Response to Levodopa

Age

The bioavailability of levodopa is greater in old than young people by a factor of 2–3. The elimination phase in plasma is however similar in young and old.

Absorption Site

Buccal

Little levodopa is absorbed at the usual oral pH of 6–6.5. Most is swallowed with saliva.

Gastric

Patients with basal acid gastric juice (pH 1.1–2.1) absorb between 5% and 23% of labelled levodopa, between 15 and 120 min after intake. In patients with gastric juice pH 6.9–7.1, absorption is negligible. There is an inverse relationship between gastric emptying time and peak serum levodopa concentration. Levodopa inhibits gastric emptying, and this is reversed by metoclopramide or domperidone, which return gastric emptying to normal. The stimulation of gastric and intestinal mobility by metoclopramide and domperidone may increase total levodopa absorption owing to rapid delivery of ingested levodopa to the small intestine.

Intestinal

The main site of absorption of levodopa is from the small bowel. Without decarboxylase inhibitors, intestinal decarboxylation of levodopa accounts for 50%–80% of an oral dose. There is an active gut transport system for levodopa in animals and probably in humans.

Diet

Dietary protein content affects the absorption of levodopa from the small intestine. Neutral amino acids compete with levodopa for the active transport mechanism across the gut wall. High protein diets (0.5 g kg^{-1} day^{-1}) may cause inhibition of levodopa absorption.

Meal Times

Meals may delay gastric emptying and delivery of levodopa to the small bowel. However, taking levodopa after meals may reduce the incidence of nausea.

Other Drugs

Anticholinergic drugs in high doses may significantly delay and also diminish the absorption of levodopa. Amantadine has little effect on the gut transport of levodopa.

Awareness of all these factors is important to determine the optimum therapeutic response to levodopa. The concurrent administration of a decarboxylase inhibitor will reduce peripheral wastage of levodopa, reduce the dosage required to elicit the therapeutic response, and decrease peripheral side effects. The combination of levodopa with domperidone (given 60 min before levodopa 10–20 mg p.o.) may very slightly enhance levodopa bioavailability and also prevent the effects of peripheral dopamine receptor stimulation, including vomiting.

Levodopa Distribution

In the plasma, more than 90% of levodopa occurs as free amino acid; less than 10% is protein bound. The plasma half-life of levodopa is approximately 1 h, and is related to the rapid distribution and metabolism of the drug. There is considerable uptake of levodopa in the gut, pancreas, liver, salivary glands, kidney and skin. Only about 5% of an oral dose reaches the brain; highest levels occur in the striatum, area postrema, median eminence and olfactory bulbs. The plasma half-life of levodopa is prolonged to 1.2–1.6 h by combination with decarboxylase inhibitor; 12–17 h after levodopa administration, blood levels remain raised.

In 40%–45% of patients given oral levodopa there are two plasma peaks as a result of initial gastric and subsequent gastrointestinal absorption. Levodopa by mouth has impaired bioavailability as compared with intravenous dosing, owing to metabolic degradation in the gut wall and multiple oral doses cause fluctuating rather than steady plasma levels. Overall, there is some correlation between levodopa dose, plasma DOPA (and plasma dopamine) level, and clinical improvement.

Despite fluctuation in plasma levels, the clinical response to levodopa given two or three times a day, or even on alternate days, is usually sustained early in the disease, but with disease progression and prolonged levodopa treatment, response fluctuations appear time-related to the plasma levodopa level. This may be due to progressive loss of dopamine storage capacity in the brain. The wearing-off phenomenon, or end-of-dose deterioration in the late stages of parkinsonism can be minimised by shortening the intervals between levodopa doses.

Long-Duration Response to Levodopa

In addition to the fundamental pharmacokinetic response to levodopa in parkinsonism with clinical benefit linked to the plasma concentration of levodopa, many patients on chronic levodopa therapy retain some clinical benefit for 3–7 days if levodopa is suddenly discontinued. The same phenomenon occurs with other antiparkinsonian drugs, anticholinergics and amantadine. Although a single dose of levodopa may cause a prolonged increase in brain neurotransmitter stores, this is unlikely to account entirely for the long-duration response to levodopa or other antiparkinsonian drugs.

Metabolism and Excretion of Dopamine

The major metabolic pathway of levodopa is decarboxylation to dopamine. The activity of released dopamine is terminated by presynaptic reuptake and enzymatic degradation. Catecholamine degradation by the extracellular enzyme catechol-*O*-methyltransferase (COMT) and the intracellular enzyme monoamine oxidase (MAO) produces homovanillic acid (HVA) in the case of dopamine, and hydroxyphenolglycol or vanillylmandelic acid (VMA) in the case of noradrenaline. These substances are acidic and reach the CSF before entering the blood. The major urinary metabolites excreted are HVA and other phenolcarboxylic acids, small quantities of dopamine, 3-*O*-methyldopa, noradrenaline metabolites, and also unchanged levodopa.

Deprenyl (Selegiline)

There are at least two monoamine oxidase isoenzymes (MAO-A and MAO-B) of which type B is predominant in the human brain. This may be inhibited by many alkaloids, cocaine, harmaline, as well as Deprenyl (selegiline). Selegiline is an MAO-B inhibitor, which, unlike MAO-A inhibitors does not produce cheese or tyramine-like reactions in total daily dosages below 30–35 mg, and can be safely combined with levodopa. In contrast, MAO-A inhibitors, given in combination with dopamine, tyramine or phenylethylamines may cause hypertension crises, as well as requiring rigid dietary restrictions. The addition of selegiline 5–10 mg daily to levodopa reduces the levodopa requirement by about 20%, and sometimes prolongs the medium-duration response to levodopa by 10–30 min. Selegiline is of most value in the treatment of late parkinsonism, and the control of dose-related response swings. Selegiline 5 mg daily causes 95% irreversible MAO-B inhibition. Selegiline is converted to amphetamine in the brain and liver, but in low doses (5–10 mg daily) amphetamine-like CNS stimulant action is not seen.

Adverse Effects of Levodopa

The adverse effects of levodopa (Table 5.6) are attributable to dopamine receptor stimulation at different sites inside and outside the CNS.

Table 5.6. Major adverse reactions to levodopa in patients with parkinsonism

Effect	Approximate frequency (%)	
	Without decarboxylase inhibitor	With decarboxylase inhibitor
Cardiovascular		
Postural hypotension		
Asymptomatic	90	40
Symptomatic	5	5
Palpitations, flushing, arrhythmia	10–20	2–5
Gastrointestinal		
Nausea and vomiting	80	15
Neuropsychiatric		
Agitation		
Anxiety	20	25
Aggression, delusions, hallucinations, etc.	20	25
Changes in mood, awareness	20	25
Involuntary movements		
Restlessness, chorea	70	80
Dystonia	10	15

The minor increase in neuropsychiatric problems and involuntary movements with levodopa–decarboxylase inhibitor combinations, compared with levodopa alone, is probably due to tolerance of higher effective levodopa dosage owing to reduction in nausea and vomiting. Decarboxylase inhibitors per se may cause hyperprolactinaemia.

Levodopa causes a fall in systolic and diastolic blood pressure because dopamine stimulates blood vessels, peripheral nerve terminals and the central nervous system. Hypotension with an average fall in systolic blood pressure of 20 mmHg occurs in most subjects given levodopa, but is usually asymptomatic. However, faintness and dizziness are not uncommon at the start of treatment, or may first occur, usually in disabled and hypokinetic subjects, 2–5 years after the start of therapy. When severe, hypotension with syncope may prevent levodopa therapy. An upright posture at night will partially reduce this side effect, and postural hypotension may be occasionally controlled with elastic stockings, oral ephedrine 30–120 mg, fludrocortisone 0.1 mg, or DDAVP (see Chap. 11).

A wide range of cardiac dysrhythmias occurs with levodopa although the incidence of transient sinus tachycardia and atrial and ventricular extrasystoles is low, and may be reduced still further by the addition of decarboxylase inhibitors or domperidone. One of these combinations should be used in parkinsonian subjects with heart disease. The benefits of levodopa in practice usually outweigh any risk of cardiac dysrhythmia.

Vomiting, with or without nausea, occurs 20–90 min after a dose of levodopa in about 80% of all subjects. Tolerance to this emetic effect occurs in most, but not all subjects after several months of treatment. Vomiting with levodopa is due to stimulation of the medullary emetic centre situated in the brain stem (but outside the blood–brain barrier to dopamine), and not to stimulation of gastric dopamine receptors. Nausea can be avoided by giving low single doses of levodopa (125–250 mg), increasing daily dosage very slowly (increments of 250–500 mg weekly), and by taking levodopa with food to slow absorption.

Combination of levodopa with decarboxylase inhibitors reduces the incidence of vomiting from approximately 80% to 15%. To achieve adequate inhibition of peripheral decarboxylation, a minimum dose of carbidopa (75 mg daily) or benserazide (100 mg) is required. In addition, or alternatively to decarboxylase inhibitors, metoclopramide 10–20 mg, domperidone 10–20 mg, or antacids may be given 30–60 min before levodopa.

Metoclopramide, but not domperidone, will penetrate the brain, and partially prevent the therapeutic response to levodopa. Other gastrointestinal side effects sometimes attributed to levodopa include constipation (although this probably results from concomitant anticholinergic drugs), diarrhoea, flatulence and heartburn. Gastrointestinal bleeding has occurred in subjects with a history of peptic ulceration given levodopa (and also bromocriptine, see p. 85).

Agitation, anxiety, elation, insomnia, drowsiness, depression, aggression, paranoid ideas, hallucinations, delusions or unmasking of dementia may occur within a few days to several years after starting levodopa, and usually occur at the time of levodopa dose increase, pyrexia, or the addition of another antiparkinsonian drug. These psychiatric disorders are common, and some degree of nocturnal confusion occurs in 20%–30% of all parkinsonian patients on levodopa. Improvement usually occurs 1–2 weeks after levodopa withdrawal. The addition of decarboxylase inhibitors to levodopa, if this permits an effective increase in levodopa dosage, tends to increase the frequency and severity of mental disturbances (see Table 5.6).

Mild psychotic symptoms, with change in mood or awareness, may be acceptable as the price of improved mobility. Levodopa-induced neuro-psychiatric disorders can be treated if necessary with a psychotropic drug or non-phenothiazine derivative such as chlormethiazole.

Insomnia, changes in sleep pattern, or daytime sleepiness occur rarely in patients on levodopa, although usually this does not alter awareness. Elevation or depression of mood has been recorded on levodopa, although this may be secondary to alteration in the severity of parkinsonism.

Levodopa dyskinesias usually occur at the same time as the greatest degree of clinical improvement, and are predominantly choreic. They occur with high DOPA plasma levels, and are usually dose-related. These peak-dose dyskinesias become more severe and disabling with the progression of both treatment and disease, although a small proportion, perhaps 10% of subjects, do not develop involuntary movements. Diphasic dyskinesias are less common, and occur in 5%–10% of all patients treated with levodopa. In contrast to peak-dose dyskinesias, diphasic dyskinesias occur at the start and at the end of action of a single levodopa dose. Reducing individual doses of levodopa should reduce peak-dose dyskinesias and increasing the dose may possibly avoid diphasic dyskinesias. However, both these techniques are usually unsatisfactory with either levodopa toxicity and constant dyskinesias at high levodopa levels, or inadequate response from a lower dosage. The alleged failure of dopamine agonist ergot derivatives such as bromocriptine to cause dyskinesias is perhaps because these drugs, however high the dose, are less potent than levodopa in the treatment of parkinsonism, and mild involuntary movements may go unnoticed.

The only satisfactory way to avoid levodopa dyskinesias is to reduce levodopa dosage or give small, but frequent (2-hourly) oral doses of levodopa if response fluctuation occurs with more widely separated doses. Constant intravenous levodopa infusion to achieve steady plasma levels will also prevent the problem, at least for a few days. The possibility of preventing dyskinesias with the selective blockade of a "dyskinesia-generating" popula-tion of dopamine receptors with neuroleptics such as tiapride or oxiperomide is of theoretical rather than practical importance. Both these drugs may induce drowsiness.

Other adverse reactions to levodopa are infrequent. Patients with chronic wide-angle glaucoma may be treated cautiously with levodopa, but this is contraindicated in patients with narrow-angle glaucoma. The hormonal consequences of levodopa are not of clinical importance in elderly parkinso-nian subjects. Polyuria, incontinence, difficulty in micturition, and retention reported with levodopa usually result from infection, other genitourinary disease or concomitant anticholinergic drugs.

Biochemical and haematological changes are minor, and include slight and usually transient rises in blood urea nitrogen, increased serum transaminases, alkaline phosphatase and bilirubin and the occurrence of a positive direct Coombs' test, but not haemolysis.

The safety of levodopa has now been demonstrated over a decade of use. No separate reactions attributable to the use of decarboxylase inhibitors have been reported in humans. Levodopa, combined with a decarboxylase inhibitor or domperidone can be given to patients with cardiac or renal disease, although there is a slight possibility of provoking atrial, nodal or ventricular dysrhythmias, particularly following myocardial infarction. Some caution is needed in the treatment of patients with active peptic ulcers. Periodic biochemical evaluation is unnecessary.

Drug Interactions with Levodopa

Levodopa may be combined with ergot derivatives, anticholinergics and amantadine, and also with analgesics, tricyclic antidepressants, antidiabetic and antihypertensive drugs. Serious adverse reactions to levodopa in combination with anaesthetics have not been reported, but if a general anaesthetic is unavoidable, levodopa should be discontinued 6 h prior to surgery. The motor effects of levodopa are diminished by phenothiazines, butyrophenones, reserpine and pyridoxine, and enhanced by anticholinergics, amphetamine, amantadine and decarboxylase inhibitors.

Indirectly Acting Dopamine Agonists

Amantadine

Amantadine inhibits catecholamine reuptake in central and peripheral neurones, and causes an increase in neurotransmitter output in response to nerve stimuli. It has CNS stimulant, antiparkinsonian, and antiviral effects. These are due to different mechanisms. Amantadine was initially used as an antiviral agent, and interferes with cell entry of RNA-containing viruses, but is of proven value in the prevention and treatment of only one viral disease in humans, influenza A_2. It is not of proven clinical value in animal scrapie, Jakob–Creutzfeldt disease, or acute sclerosing leucoencephalitis. The multiplication of various influenza virus strains is inhibited by adrenaline and noradrenaline, ammonium salts and halogenophenylethylamines as well as amantadine.

Amantadine does not alter motor activity in normal people. However, in 1968, a woman with parkinsonism treated with amantadine for influenza prophylaxis reported a remarkable improvement in tremor, rigidity and akinesia. This serendipitous observation was followed by the report that amantadine improved two-thirds of patients with Parkinson's disease, although a small percentage develop tolerance after 6–12 weeks' treatment. Overall, amantadine 100–300 mg daily gives a little greater improvement than anticholinergics, much less than levodopa. A quarter of patients report CNS stimulant effects, jitteriness, insomnia, vertigo and loss of appetite. There are two reports of patients developing epilepsy during high-dose amantadine treatment (600–800 mg daily), and like all antiparkinsonian drugs, amantadine may produce alteration in awareness and hallucinosis. Livedo reticularis develops in 30%–50% of all subjects, and ankle oedema in 15%, with no signs of cardiac, liver or renal disease. These changes are dose-related, and reversible 2–6 weeks after amantadine withdrawal. Amantadine does not cause dyskinesias.

Amantadine is a symmetrical primary amine, and is well absorbed after oral administration; it is not metabolised in humans, but excreted unchanged in the urine. Amantadine is sparingly soluble and may be given i.v., but there is an appreciable risk of venous thrombosis. The analogue rimantadine and amantadine spiro compounds have similar properties. Amantadine is chemically a base and completely absorbed from the intestine rather than the stomach. Maximum plasma levels occur 1–4 h after a single oral dose, with a half-life of 10–30 h. Steady state plasma concentrations are achieved after a few days' treatment.

Therapeutic plasma levels on amantadine 300 mg daily are 0.68–1.0 mg/l. Toxic overdose of amantadine (2.1 g) has been described in a single patient. Signs of parkinsonism were completely abolished at the expense of severe confusion, hallucinations and hyperpyrexia. Spontaneous recovery occurred in 4 days.

Directly Acting Dopamine Agonists

Many drugs which mimic the action of levodopa, including apomorphine, norpropylnoraporphine, piribedil, and different ergot derivatives have been used to treat Parkinson's disease. These drugs have important pharmacological differences from levodopa, but cause broadly similar clinical responses. Overall, they are less effective than levodopa. In contrast, the ergot derivatives are of greater value than levodopa in the treatment of hyperprolactinaemia and acromegaly.

Bromocriptine

This lysergic acid derivative is a weak base, insoluble in water. The addition of the bromine atom in position 2 changes the pharmacological actions of the compound, and increases dopamine-stimulant effects. In spite of being an ergot derivative it is remarkably free of vascular side effects.

Bromocriptine is available as the methanesulphonate (mesylate). The drug is rapidly and completely absorbed from the gastrointestinal tract, and does not greatly alter gastric mobility. Vomiting, as with levodopa, is due to a central rather than a peripheral side effect of bromocriptine. The central effects indicate that bromocriptine penetrates most areas of the brain.

Peak plasma levels of 4–20 ng/ml occur 2–3 h after oral doses of 12.5–100 mg. Optimum peak plasma bromocriptine levels in Parkinson's disease are usually between 2 and 5 ng parent drug per millilitre plasma. High plasma levels remain for several hours and very low levels can be detected in the plasma for up to 4 days. The plasma time–concentration curve corresponds fairly well with motor activation and prolactin suppression. Improvement in parkinsonism with bromocriptine is dose-related, low doses (5–20 mg daily) giving perhaps similar benefit to the anticholinergic drug orphenadrine hydrochloride 150 mg daily, although high dosages are rarely as effective as optimum levodopa doses.

Bromocriptine is metabolised extensively with at least 30 excretory products, owing to isomerisation and hydrolysis of the lysergic acid part of the molecule and oxidation of the peptide fragment. Excretion of bromocriptine metabolites is mainly biliary, and about 70% appears in the faeces over 5 days after a single oral dose of 2.5 mg. A small part of the dose, 6%–7% is excreted unchanged or as metabolites in the urine.

The initial bromocriptine dose should not exceed 1–1.25 mg. This low dose may rarely cause severe collapse with rapid recovery. Dose increases should not be greater than 2.5–5 mg on alternate days, so that it can take 1 month to achieve therapeutic levels in acromegaly and 3 months in Parkinson's disease.

Bromocriptine in Parkinson's Disease

Bromocriptine is superior to levodopa in the treatment of hormonal disorders, but not of Parkinson's disease, owing to differences in drug access to the pituitary and basal ganglia, as well as to differences in agonist activity at the two sites. Reduction of dopamine stores in late parkinsonism may also limit the action of bromocriptine. Overall, bromocriptine 10–20 mg has about the same effect as levodopa 100 mg combined with a decarboxylase inhibitor.

In some patients the combination of both drugs gives better results than bromocriptine alone. Despite a lower potency, bromocriptine has a more prolonged action than levodopa, and the incidence of side effects is different. Patients with dose-related response swings on levodopa often achieve a more stable response with the addition of bromocriptine 5–20 mg 6- to 8-hourly.

Bromocriptine causes choreic and dystonic movements identical to those produced by levodopa, but much less frequently. Vomiting is infrequent, so bromocriptine may be a satisfactory alternative when levodopa causes persistent nausea, despite the addition of decarboxylase inhibitors and antiemetics. On the other hand, bromocriptine causes altered behaviour and awareness more often than levodopa. These disturbances can last from 2 to 6 weeks after bromocriptine withdrawal. Like levodopa, bromocriptine causes a slight and usually asymptomatic fall in blood pressure in upright and recumbent patients. Raynaud's phenomenon, erythromelalgia and livedo reticularis sometimes occur.

Other Ergot Derivatives

Lisuride is soluble and may be given i.v. It has a very rapid duration of action, 1–2 h, and peak effects occur 15–30 min following administration of lisuride 0.15 mg i.v. Clinical actions and side effects are similar to levodopa, with the exception that lisuride often causes sedation, and may sometimes be effective in the treatment of dystonia. The dopamine receptor stimulant effect of pergolide, unlike bromocriptine, is independent of dopamine stores. Pergolide is the longest-acting ergot derivative so far investigated in parkinsonism, although motor effects (6–8 h) are shorter than hormonal effects (prolactin suppression for 24–36 h). Table 5.7 compares the effects of levodopa, amantadine, bromocriptine, pergolide and lisuride.

Treatment of Parkinson's Disease

The various antiparkinsonian drugs (anticholinergics, amantadine, levodopa, selegiline and ergot drugs all have a role in treating the illness, but are employed at different stages of the disease.

The Newly Diagnosed Case

At this stage, disability is likely to be mild to moderate. With the possible exception of selegiline (see later discussion), none of the antiparkinsonian drugs affects the progression of the underlying pathology of Parkinson's disease; they are symptomatic, not curative therapies. Accordingly, these drugs do not have to be given the moment the diagnosis is made.

Selegiline may be the exception, for there are theoretical reasons, but very little definite evidence, to suggest that inhibition of MAO-B activity might conceivably slow the rate of progression of Parkinson's disease. The theory is based on the understanding of the mode of toxicity of the agent MPTP (1-methyl-4-phenyl-1,2,3,6-tetrahydropyridine), which has caused dramatic subacute parkinsonism in young drug addicts in California. MPTP was an inadvertant contaminant of a synthetic "designer drug" produced by illicit chemists as a substitute for narcotics. Within days of exposure to MPTP, some addicts developed all the signs of Parkinson's disease. Subsequently, they have been treated successfully with levodopa.

MPTP turns out to be a highly selective neurotoxin, producing destruction of the pigmented cells of the substantia nigra, which is the core pathology of Parkinson's disease itself. Thus, MPTP represents an environmental toxin that can cause both the clinical symptoms and pathology of Parkinson's disease. Since Parkinson's disease itself is not hereditary (the incidence in identical twins is similar to that in nonidentical twins), there is speculation that it may be due to exposure to environmental toxins similar to MPTP.

Table 5.7. Comparative effects of levodopa, amantadine, bromocriptine, pergolide and lisuride

Effect	Levodopa	Amantadine	Bromocriptine	Pergolide	Lisuride
Pharmacological action	Increase in dopamine synthesis	Increase in dopamine release	Presynaptic and postsynaptic receptor stimulation	Postsynaptic receptor agonist	Postsynaptic receptor agonist
Total daily dose					
Hyperprolactinaemia	Not used	Not used	5–10 mg	1–2 mg	2.4–5 mg
Acromegaly	Not used	Not used	20–60 mg	2–4 mg	2.4–5 mg
Parkinson's disease	0.5–4 g	100–300 mg	20–120 mg	2–8 mg	1 mg
Duration of action of single dose	1–4 h	4–6 h	4–8 h	6–12 h	2–4 h
Hormonal effects	Variable and brief	Minor, although potentiates levodopa	Potent and sustained	Potent and sustained	Potent and sustained
Motor effects	Most potent antiparkinsonian drug available	Minor symptomatic improvement, no dyskinesias	Less potent than levodopa	Less potent than levodopa, although response prolonged	Can be given as infusion
Vascular actions	Fall in blood pressure, in renal blood flow, cardiac arrhythmias	Livedo reticularis	As levodopa, Raynaud's phenomenon, erythromelalgia	As bromocriptine	As levodopa
Emesis	Common, but minimised by decarboxylase inhibitors or domperidone	Rare	Uncommon; very rare in puerperal women	Uncommon	Uncommon
Disorders of awareness and behaviour, hallucinations	20%–30% of patients	Uncommon in 100–300 mg daily dosage	Dose- and age-related, may persist for 2–6 weeks	As bromocriptine	As levodopa

The way in which MPTP destroys the substantia nigra has been worked out in experimental studies. MPTP causes parkinsonism and nigral damage in nonhuman primates. MPTP itself is not the toxic agent; once it reaches the brain it is converted into MPP^+ by the action of MAO-B in glia. MPP^+ is then taken up into nigral neurones by the dopamine uptake system; MPP^+ then binds to neuromelanin in nigral nerve cells, where it is trapped, and MPP^+ kills these nerve cells by generation of free radicals and interference with energy metabolism. This remarkable series of events can be prevented at a number of points. Inhibitors of MAO-B, such as selegiline; inhibitors of dopamine uptake, such as mazindol (see Chap. 7); and free radical scavengers all may prevent the neurotoxicity of MPTP. So if Parkinson's disease is due to continual exposure to something like MPTP, then early treatment with an MAO-B inhibitor such as selegiline, might at least in theory, slow progression of the disease.

Returning to the practical management of the early case of Parkinson's disease, recently diagnosed, the question is which, if any of the symptomatic antiparkinsonian therapies should be employed first. If disability is very mild, no drug treatment may be required to begin with. However, the disease is progressive and sooner or later some form of treatment will be necessary.

Levodopa is the most effective antiparkinsonian drug, but it has been suggested that there may be reasons for delaying its introduction. Levodopa therapy often becomes less effective after some years of treatment. Levodopa-induced dyskinesias and fluctuations in the response emerge with time or with disease progression. Accordingly, it may be wise to employ other drugs to begin with, reserving levodopa for later.

Mild early cases may be adequately controlled by anticholinergics and/or amantadine for some time. Anticholinergics were the earliest treatment for Parkinson's disease, but there are some reservations to their use, particularly in the elderly, who are very prone to develop mental side effects on these drugs.

If disability cannot be relieved by anticholinergics and/or amantadine, or if it is severe from the beginning, then levodopa is required. Bromocriptine is not usually as effective when given by itself; only about a third of patients can be managed on bromocriptine alone.

Accordingly, when disability demands it, levodopa is introduced in combination with a peripheral decarboxylase inhibitor (to reduce initial nausea and vomiting), in the form of Sinemet or Madopar. There is little to choose between these two formulations. The drugs are given after food in gradually increasing dosage until disability is controlled. If nausea and vomiting prove a problem, each dose of Sinemet or Madopar can be prefaced by domperidone (10–20 mg 1 h before levodopa administration). Anticholinergics and/or amantadine, if started earlier, can be continued with levodopa.

The Early Years

To begin with, levodopa therapy produces a sustained smooth response. Drug intake three or four times a day usually provides continuous relief of symptoms. Side effects due to levodopa overdosage, such as dyskinesias and mental disturbances, may occur, but disappear if the dose of levodopa is reduced. If the patient develops confusion, hallucinations or psychosis, concurrent anti-cholinergics and amantadine should be gradually withdrawn first, after a search for some intercurrent infection or other illness which may precipitate such mental changes, particularly in the elderly. The aim in each individual is to titrate the daily dose of Sinemet or Madopar to that which provides adequate relief of symptoms, with minimal or no side effects.

With the passage of time, however, a considerable proportion of patients (approximately 50% after 5 years treatment) begin to develop fluctuations in their response to levodopa therapy. They begin to notice that the benefit from each dose lasts for a shorter period of time—the effect of each dose wears off earlier and earlier (end-of-dose deterioration). The patient then swings from mobility (usually with dyskinesias) to immobility at intervals throughout the day, related in time to each dose of levodopa. Such swings often become more and more abrupt, until they occur within minutes (on–off phenomenon).

Management of the Fluctuating Patient

The first step in overcoming a fluctuating response to therapy in those on long-term treatment is to rearrange the schedule of levodopa treatment; smaller doses are required at shorter intervals. Many patients now require Sinemet or Madopar every 2–3 h throughout the day. They also may need an extra dose during the night to overcome nocturnal akinesia. The duration of action of each dose of levodopa should be established in each patient, and the drug given at that appropriate interval. The size of each dose is titrated to achieve maximum mobility with minimum side effects.

If this approach does not achieve smooth control, then selegiline is added. The latter slightly prolongs the duration of action of each dose of levodopa. However, this approach often only produces limited improvement, so the next stage is to introduce bromocriptine in addition to levodopa. The latter is continued at the usual frequency, as bromocriptine is added, beginning with a small single dose, and gradually increasing over a matter of weeks. At the same time the dosage (but not timing) of levodopa will have to be reduced to prevent increasing dyskinesias and mental side effects. The aim is to replace about one-third to one-half of levodopa intake with bromocriptine.

Unfortunately, these measures may not provide constant relief of parkinson-ism in some patients. Newer methods are being explored to overcome the problem of severe fluctuations in levodopa response, including long-acting forms of the drug, and continuous subcutaneous delivery of a dopamine agonist such as lisuride by minipump.

Dyskinesias and Mental Side Effects

These represent the two major adverse effects of levodopa therapy. Both are dose-dependent, but unfortunately reducing levodopa dosage to get rid of them often leads to an unacceptable return of parkinsonian disability. Many patients may accept some degree of dyskinesia in return for relief of parkinsonism. Peak-dose choreiform dyskinesias generally are not painful, although they are unsightly. No other drugs are available to reduce their severity without worsening parkinsonism. Dystonic dyskinesias, which often occur at the beginning and/or end of dose (diphasic dyskinesias), and early morning dystonia, however, may be very painful. Early morning dystonia may be helped by taking a dose of levodopa during the night, or by a dose of a longer-acting dopamine agonist last thing at night. Diphasic dyskinesias may be eased by increasing the frequency of levodopa intake to overlap individual doses, but often this produces unacceptable peak-dose dyskinesias. Lithium sometimes helps painful dystonic dyskinesias.

Mental problems are unfortunately a common problem in Parkinson's disease. About 20% of patients, especially the elderly, may become demented, with progression of their disease. In others the mental changes may be due to intercurrent illness or drugs. Unfortunately, the agents required to control confusion, paranoia, hallucinations, psychosis or aggression frequently cause worsening of the parkinsonism. Every attempt should be made to identify some infective or other cause, to withdraw anticholinergic drugs and amantadine, and then to reduce levodopa (or bromocriptine) dosage to the lowest level compatible with acceptable mobility. If mental problems persist, and are disturbing, it may occasionally be necessary to add a sedative such as heminevrin or a benzodiazepine, or even a neuroleptic such as thioridazine although the latter may aggravate the parkinsonism.

Depression is a common problem in Parkinson's disease, often requiring treatment. Around a third of patients will complain of depression, which is generally related to the severity of physical disability. Relief of parkinsonian symptoms may improve depression, but specific antidepressant drug therapy is often required. Tricyclic and tetracyclic antidepressants, such as amitriptyline, can be used with levodopa, although their anticholinergic actions may summate with those of specific antiparkinsonian anticholinergic drugs. MAO-A inhibitors can not be used with levodopa.

Treatment of Chorea and Ballism

Chorea and hemiballism may be reduced by dopamine antagonists (see p. 94). Drugs acting presynaptically to deplete dopamine stores (tetrabenazine 75–150 mg/day), or postsynaptically to block dopamine receptors (phenothiazines such as chlorpromazine 75–300 mg/day, butyrophenones such as haloperidol 1.5–2.0 mg/day, or substituted benzamides such as sulpiride 600–1200 mg/day) may be effective. The dose is increased gradually until control of chorea is achieved, or side effects intrude. All these drugs cause parkinsonism, and tetrabenazine in particular may produce depression. Often the threshold between control of chorea and drug-induced parkinsonism is very finely balanced. Indeed, many patients find that side effects outweigh the benefits of improvement of chorea, and prefer not to take drugs. However, neuroleptics may also be required to control the behavioural disturbances that occur in Huntington's disease.

Hemiballism, which usually is due to a stroke in an elderly diabetic hypertensive patient, tends to recover spontaneously over some months. But initially the wild abnormal movements may be very distressing and sometimes even lead to death. They can be controlled by tetrabenazine or haloperidol in nearly every case, but rarely require stereotactic thalamotomy.

Treatment of Tics

Most minor tics require no treatment, but severe tics and particularly those of Gilles de la Tourette syndrome may require therapy. The vocalisations and obscenities that characterise the latter disease may cause considerable distress to the embarrassed child or adolescent. The severity of Gilles de la Tourette syndrome waxes and wanes, so that treatment may be necessary only for limited periods. Neuroleptics such as haloperidol or sulpiride may reduce tics and vocalisations, but there are problems in their use. All neuroleptics have the propensity to cause parkinsonism and tardive dyskinesias (see p. 94), and may interfere with concentration and learning. Gilles de la Tourette syndrome begins in childhood, but is usually a lifelong illness, so the decision to treat is committing the individual to long-term neuroleptic therapy. It is best to reserve such treatment for those in whom the illness is causing severe social disability, and to review the need for continuation of drugs at regular intervals. The noradrenergic α_2 agonist clonidine also may reduce tics in some patients, and is an alternative therapy.

Treatment of Dystonia

Patients with dystonia are often disabled by their muscle spasms. Unfortunately, they do not respond uniformly to any one class of drugs, but the most effective are the anticholinergics. Children with dystonia often progress to generalised disease. A small subset, often characterised by diurnal fluctuations of their illness (better in the morning and after sleep), respond rapidly and dramatically to small doses of levodopa (as Sinemet or Madopar), which should be tried first. If there is no benefit from levodopa within 3 months, it can be withdrawn, and an anticholinergic such as benzhexol should be started. About 50% of children with dystonia gain benefit from benzhexol, but very large doses (40–100 mg/day) may be required. The aim is to introduce benzhexol in low dosage (2–5 mg daily) and increase very slowly by about 2–5 mg/day at 1- or 2-weekly intervals. The dose is gradually increased until adequate relief is achieved or side effects (dry mouth, blurred vision, urinary difficulties, memory and behavioural disturbances or frank toxic confusional states) intrude. Other drugs that may help a few patients include benzodiazepines, baclofen and carbamazepine.

Adults usually present with a focal dystonia (blepharospasm, Meige's syndrome, spasmodic torticollis, or dystonic writer's cramp) which does not progress. As in children, anticholinergic drugs are the most effective therapy, but the response is less predictable, with only about 30% gaining benefit; side effects are more likely, especially in the elderly.

Because drug treatment frequently fails to control dystonia, other methods of therapy may be employed. Blepharospasm causing functional blindness can be relieved by injection of botulinus toxin into the periocular muscles to cause local weakness. This method restores vision in 70% of cases, but the injections have to be repeated every 2–3 months, as recovery occurs owing to terminal sprouting. Open surgery to section the branches of the facial nerve to the orbicularis oculi may be required in those who fail to respond to botulinus toxin.

A number of surgical treatments have been devised for spasmodic torticollis, but most of these (stereotactic thalamotomy and division of the upper cervical motor roots at laminectomy) have fallen out of favour. However, selective extraspinal division of the posterior primary rami of the upper cervical nerves, combined with division of the spinal accessory nerve, may be successful in those severely disabled by torticollis or retrocollis.

Stereotactic surgery has a place in the treatment of hemidystonia. A unilateral thalamotomy contralateral to the affected limbs, carries only a 1% risk of hemiplegia and can be effective. Bilateral thalamotomy, however, is less successful for generalised dystonia, and produces severe disruption of speech in 20% of cases.

Treatment of Tremor

Tremor in Parkinson's disease often responds to the usual treatment of that condition, although less reliably than akinesia and rigidity. The postural tremor of essential (familial) tremor often responds dramatically to alcohol (for unknown reasons), but this is not often a practical therapy. Two other classes of drugs may help essential tremor, beta-adrenergic antagonists and barbiturates. Propranolol (30–240 mg/day) reduces essential tremor in about 60% of cases. Primidone (375–1000 mg/day) is also of benefit in about the same proportion. Unfortunately, no drugs reliably help the disabling cerebellar tremor that may occur in those with multiple sclerosis or cerebellar degenerations.

Treatment of Myoclonus

Many types of myoclonus arise from abnormal electrical discharges in the cerebral cortex, so are related to epilepsy and are treated with anticonvulsants. Sodium valproate and clonazepam (see Chap. 4) are the most effective antimyoclonic agents. Often they are given together for maximum benefit. Some types of myoclonus, particularly that which follows cerebral anoxia, may respond to treatment with the serotonin precursor 5-hydroxytryptophan with a peripheral decarboxylase inhibitor.

Drug-Induced Movement Disorders

Many drugs cause abnormal movement (Table 5.8). Of particular importance are the range of movement disorders produced by neuroleptic drugs. Neuroleptic drugs (phenothiazines, butyrophenones, diphenylbutylpiperidines, thioxanthenes and substituted benzamides) are widely employed to control psychiatric illnesses such as schizophrenia. However, they are also used to treat vertigo and nausea (e.g. prochlorperazine), and a range of gastrointestinal disorders (e.g. metoclopramide). They may cause movement disorders in any of these conditions.

All neuroleptics, of whatever class, may cause drug-induced parkinsonism, which generally is dose-dependent although it occurs more commonly in the elderly. Drug-induced parkinsonism has all the clinical features of Parkinson's disease. Anticholinergics are usually employed to combat drug-induced parkinsonism if neuroleptics have to be continued, as for schizophrenia. If neuroleptic drugs can be withdrawn, drug-induced parkinsonism nearly always remits, although it may take months or a year or so to disappear.

Acute dystonic reactions to neuroleptic drugs are uncommon, but are frequently misdiagnosed. They usually occur within a few days of starting neuroleptic treatment, and can be rapidly reduced by an intravenous injection of an anticholinergic drug or benzodiazepine.

Akathisia (an unpleasant sense of motor restlessness accompanied by an uncontrollable desire to move) often accompanies acute dystonic reactions, drug-induced parkinsonism or tardive dyskinesia. It may respond to propranolol or a benzodiazepine.

Tardive dyskinesias are the most disturbing of the drug-induced dyskinesias, for they may not remit when neuroleptics are withdrawn. They appear after months or years of therapy, or may occur when neuroleptics are stopped or their dosage reduced (withdrawal dyskinesias). Overall, tardive dyskinesias appear in about 20% of those on chronic neuroleptic treatment.

The commonest tardive dyskinesia is an abnormal movement of the mouth, tongue and jaw (tardive buccolingual masticatory dyskinesia). This is particularly common in the elderly, and resembles a similar condition that may

Table 5.8. Drug-induced movement disorders

Disorder	Drugs responsible	Susceptible age group	Prevalence	Onset after initiation of therapy	Effect of withdrawal of drug	Treatment
Tremor	Bronchodilators, Tricyclics, Lithium carbonate, Caffeine, Amphetamine	Any	Dose-dependent, about 35%	Rapid	Disappears	Withdraw drug
Parkinsonism	Reserpine, Tetrabenazine, Neuroleptics	Any, but increases with age	Dose-dependent, about 50%	Gradual within first few months	Disappears slowly, may take 1 year	Anticholinergics
Acute dystonia	Neuroleptics, Diazoxide	Children, (young) adults	2%–5%	Acute within first few hours or days	Disappears	Anticholinergics, Diazepam
Akathisia	Neuroleptics	Any	About 30%	Gradual, within first few months	Disappears	Anticholinergics, Propranolol, Diazepam
Tardive dyskinesia	Neuroleptics	Increases with age	About 20%	Delayed, but increases	May get worse, persists in about 40%	Withdraw drug, tetrabenazine

occur spontaneously in that age group. However, it is about five times more common in those on neuroleptic drugs. Tardive dystonia, which resembles spontaneous dystonia, is more prevalent in younger patients on neuroleptics.

Treatment is difficult. If possible, the offending drugs should be stopped, but this may not be possible in those with active schizophrenia, who have a high risk of relapse of their psychosis. If neuroleptics can be withdrawn, tardive dyskinesias disappear in about 60% of cases, but may take months or even up to 5 years to do so.

Unfortunately, there are no effective drugs to control tardive dyskinesias. Anticholinergics make the buccolingual masticatory syndrome worse, but may help tardive dystonias. Increasing the dose of neuroleptic may help initially, but is irrational. Tetrabenazine may be of benefit, but often causes depression, which is a serious risk in schizophrenia.

Multiple Sclerosis

In any discussion of multiple sclerosis, the section on treatment is usually the shortest. However, despite the absence of definitive treatment or cure, much can be done by the careful use of drugs to help the patient, particularly with bladder control (Chap. 10), pain (Chap. 2), depression, and spasticity (see the following section).

The diagnosis of multiple sclerosis in established disease is usually not difficult. Useful confirmation is given by the finding of abnormally delayed cortical, brain stem or spinal cord evoked potentials, showing subclinical involvement. Clinically silent lesions may also be revealed by CT and nuclear magnetic resonance scans. In the late disease, oligoclonal immunoglobulins are found in the cerebrospinal fluid in over 90% of patients, although this finding is not specific for multiple sclerosis.

Spasticity

Spasticity is often best left untreated in a mobile patient. Some patients rely on their extensor hypotonus, and reducing this with drugs may increase rather than reduce disability. A number of drugs are available for the treatment of chronic severe spasticity resulting from multiple sclerosis, stroke, spinal cord injury, cerebral palsy and other disorders. These drugs are of value when spasticity is so severe that increased muscular resistance to stretch, clonus or exaggerated reflex posturing interfere with the activities of daily living such as exercise, posture, equilibrium, walking, transfer manoeuvres, or the use of braces. Skeletal muscle relaxants, with the exception of dantrolene, act primarily on the central nervous system, brain stem and spinal cord. These drugs are effective in most forms of spasticity, although treatment of provoking factors such as infection and pressure sores is fundamental.

Muscle spasm is sometimes managed more successfully by combinations of benzodiazepines, dantrolene, baclofen and cyproheptadine, than by one drug alone. However, a single drug should be used in initial treatment. It must be realised that the therapeutic goal is usually very limited.

Benzodiazepines (Chap. 7) have muscle relaxant effects mainly in proportion to their anxiolytic and hypnotic actions. Spasticity therefore is usually only relieved at the expense of some sedation. There is probably little to choose between different benzodiazepines, although compounds with a long half-life are probably of most value in the management of chronic spasticity. Diazepam is commonly used, but other benzodiazepines, clorazepate and medazepam, may be worth a trial.

Baclofen, in slowly increasing doses from 5 mg three times daily to 100 mg a day, given in divided doses, is an alternative to benzodiazepines, with a comparable clinical effect, acting at the spinal level to reduce muscle tone. Like benzodiazepines, baclofen may cause drowsiness, confusion and fatigue. In the treatment of the rare stiff-man syndrome, benzodiazepines are probably more effective than baclofen.

Dantrolene acts directly on skeletal muscle, but also has a central effect, as shown by the drowsiness, dizziness and enhancement of effect of other central nervous system depressants that dantrolene causes. Patience is needed to titrate the best dose, and the full effect of dantrolene can take several weeks to establish. Initial dantrolene oral dosage is 25 mg daily, slowly increased over 7 weeks to a maximum of 100 mg four times daily. A few cases of jaundice in patients receiving dantrolene have been reported, and liver function should be tested before, and 6 weeks after, starting treatment in all patients. If liver function tests are abnormal, dantrolene should not be commenced or should be stopped. As with all these drugs, patients should be advised not to drive a motor vehicle, or do potentially dangerous work, until therapy has been stabilised.

Impaired Bladder Control

Frequency, urgency and incontinence of micturition are common distressing problems in multiple sclerosis. Urodynamic studies may help to decide the underlying mechanism. Anticholinergic drugs (see Chap. 10) may improve symptoms due to an unstable detrusor muscle. If bladder neck obstruction is present, alpha-adrenergic blockade with prazosin or phenoxybenzamine is sometimes helpful. It is rarely necessary to consider bladder neck surgery or ileal conduit diversion. Urinary tract infection should be treated with antibiotics, except in catheterised patients, where antibiotics are best avoided unless the infection is complicated by septicaemia.

Paroxysmal Symptoms

Facial pain, unilateral ataxia, dysarthria or vertigo may appear in brief paroxysms lasting several minutes in multiple sclerosis. These symptoms are attributed to nonsynaptic transmission between axons in the presence of demyelination. Carbamazepine 100 mg three times daily sometimes prevents these symptoms.

Relapse and Prophylaxis

Most neurologists give prednisolone 60 mg daily or ACTH at the start of acute episodes of multiple sclerosis, particularly optic neuritis, and then reduce the dose gradually over 2–6 weeks. High-dosage intravenous methylprednisolone (Chap. 11) has also been used, and may result in a reduction of early disability, although this carries all the risks of steroid therapy, with occasional femoral head necrosis as well as acute allergic response.

Long-term ACTH or oral corticosteroid treatment does not alter the frequency of relapses or the rate of progression of multiple sclerosis. Many trials of immunosuppressant therapy using single or combined treatment with azathioprine, cyclophosphamide, prednisolone, anti-lymphocyte serum, and plasma exchange, have been reported, but on the whole results have been disappointing. Recent American trials of Copolymer, and attempts to immunise against the development of further episodes, may be more promising than immunosuppressant therapy.

Further Reading

Marsden CD, Fahn S (eds) (1982) Movement disorders. Neurology 2. Butterworths, London

6 Drug Treatment of Infections of the Nervous System

Bacterial Meningitis

Treatment of Meningitis

Infections of the nervous system are most common with crowding, poverty, malnutrition, or immune paresis such as accompanies malignant diseases, AIDS or the use of immunosuppressive drugs. As a general rule, the earlier the diagnosis and treatment, the better is the outcome. The mortality and morbidity from these potentially curable conditions remain unacceptably high, especially in neonatal meningitis and pneumococcal meningitis in people over 60.

A successful outcome in bacterial meningitis is largely determined by early high-dosage treatment with an antibiotic to which the infecting organism is sensitive, but is also dependent on treatment of systemic factors, with meticulous patient care, a good airway, adequate ventilation as determined by blood gas studies, the use of central venous and arterial pressure lines, fluid and electrolyte maintenance, and reduction of elevated intracranial pressure, e.g. with mannitol. A fatal outcome is associated with late diagnosis, inadequate treatment, overwhelming infection, or immune paresis. The patient may die within a few hours of the start of infection, or be left mentally handicapped, epileptic, blind, deaf or spastic. Although there has been a continuous development of new antibiotics since the introduction of penicillin, in many instances of bacterial meningitis meticulous patient care is more important than use of the latest antibiotic.

It is important to remember that inflammation of the meninges often spreads to the underlying brain, and a number of other pathological processes occur in acute meningitis, resulting in seizures and coma, as well as signs of focal brain damage. Late blockage of the normal cerebrospinal fluid pathways may cause hydrocephalus requiring a shunt. Systemic infection or toxicity is vital to recognise, and particularly common, with meningococcal and staphylococcal infections, resulting in septicaemia, circulatory collapse and renal failure.

Predisposing Factors to Meningitis

Predisposing factors to acute bacterial meningitis can be identified in most adult patients. These include:

1. Closed as well as open head injury; in particular basal skull fractures and defects in the cribriform plate; here meningitis is usually due to pneumococci, and occurs within 2 weeks of injury.

2. Neglected sinusitis, mastoiditis and otitis media are other common antecedents, and congenital spinal or skull anomalies are sometimes found; here meningitis is usually due to Gram-negative enteric bacteria, streptococci or staphylococci.

3. Immunosuppression, as in: (a) renal failure (infection with fungi or hospital pathogens, staphylococci or streptococci, particularly with dialysis); (b) cancer (cryptococci or other fungi); (c) DXT/chemotherapy (a wide range of common and uncommon pathogens); and (d) AIDS (toxoplasma, cryptococcus, fungal infections).

Diagnosis

The clinical diagnosis of meningitis must be confirmed by examining the cerebrospinal fluid and by blood culture. This should give a bacterial diagnosis, antibiotic sensitivities and measurement of cerebrospinal fluid cell, protein and sugar content.

Epidemiology

Acute pyogenic meningitis is the most common infection of the central nervous system in the United Kingdom. Most cases of bacterial meningitis are caused by meningococcus, pneumococcus, and *Hemophilus influenzae*, other forms being relatively uncommon. In children, the usual cause is *H. influenzae* or *Neisseria meningitidis*; in adults, the pneumococcus in the United Kingdom, *H. influenzae* in America and Australia. There are approximately 2000 cases of *H. influenzae* meningitis in Britain annually, with about 200 deaths.

Choice of Antibiotic (Table 6.1)

The choice of antibiotic therapy in meningitis depends on the isolation of the causative organism, and the known or predicted antibiotic sensitivity which

Table 6.1. Treatment of bacterial and fungal meningitis

Organism	Antibiotic of choice	Alternative
Pneumococcus	Benzylpenicillin or amoxycillin	Chloramphenicol
Meningococcus	Benzylpenicillin or amoxycillin	Chloramphenicol
H. influenzae	Amoxycillin plus chloramphenicol	Chloramphenicol
Escherichia coli	Amoxycillin	
Staphylococcus aureus	Benzylpenicillin or cloxacillin	Vancomycin
Mycobacterium tuberculosis	Rifampicin plus ethambutol plus isoniazid plus pyrazinamide	
Cryptococcus neoformans	Amphotericin B plus flucytosine	

must be determined in all cases. However, it is usually possible to assess the correct antibiotic from the clinical presentation before sensitivities are known.

Despite the advent of new antibiotics:

1. Penicillin and chloramphenicol remain the mainstay of initial antimicrobial treatment of acute meningitis until the organism and sensitivities are known.

2. Gentamicin also has a place, particularly in neonates. Young infants with meningitis of undetermined cause are likely to have *H. influenzae* infection. Bacterial β-lactamase production makes some of these cases resistant to penicillin.

3. Amoxycillin or benzylpenicillin must thus be combined with gentamicin for initial treatment here.

4. If Gram-negative bacteria are subsequently found resistant to these drugs, chloramphenicol is probably the treatment of choice.

5. Metronidazole is increasingly used, particularly in brain abscess, where anaerobic bacteria are common. Most of these are also sensitive to penicillin or chloramphenicol, but once an intracranial pyogenic abscess is established, this needs surgical evacuation.

Prophylaxis of Meningitis

Meningitis case-contact recognition is vital. The overall risk of meningitis in a household with *H. influenzae* or *N. meningitidis* infection is 600 times as great as in the general population of similar age. Schoolmates or hospital personnel other than those directly breathed on by the patient are not, however, at risk.

Rifampicin 600 mg for 2 days in adults, or the broad-spectrum tetracycline minocycline 100 mg twice daily for 5 days, reduced dose in children, are effective prophylaxis against *N. meningitidis*. Vaccination of *H. influenzae* contacts has been attempted, but is not very effective, with only poor protection in children younger than 2 years.

Antibiotic dosage, although determined by age, weight and renal function, must always be high in meningitis, and intravenous rather than oral therapy should be given at the start of treatment. Intrathecal drugs are rarely essential, only in those cases of resistant enteric bacteria or staphylococcal infection in which systemic therapy is not curative. Preservative-free drugs must be used for intrathecal administration, and the possibility of encephalopathy, seizures, myelitis, arachnoiditis or other complication considered.

Duration of Treatment

A single antibiotic dose may kill all infecting organisms, but it is usual to continue treatment in acute meningitis for at least 5–10 days, longer in pneumococcal and Gram-negative meningitis, since the relapse rate is high. Cerebrospinal fluid findings, rather than the clinical condition, should determine the length of treatment. Systemic antibiotic therapy should be continued for at least 5 days after the cerebrospinal fluid has become sterile.

Meningococcal Meningitis

Meningococcal meningitis is the commonest form of acute bacterial meningitis in Britain, and affects all age groups, with a high mortality in infants and the elderly.

Clinical Picture

The usual picture of acute meningococcal meningitis in a child or young adult is the rapid development over 1–2 days of fever, reduced alertness and meningism, sometimes with a petechial or purpuric rash. Infants may present with generalised seizures and fever, without localising signs. Lumbar puncture should be done before treatment is started. A definitive bacterial diagnosis, with intracellular and extracellular Gram-negative cocci, is usually possible except in patients who have received antibacterial treatment before admission. If the clinical picture fits, despite negative cerebrospinal fluid findings, penicillin or amoxycillin must be given.

Complications

In the adrenal type, with characteristic features of grave hypotension and cyanosis, the onset may be catastrophic, with disseminated intravascular coagulation (see p. 39). If laboratory facilities allow early diagnosis of disseminated intravascular coagulation (DIC), before signs of meningitis are obvious, heparin may be of value, but heparin increases the risk of haemorrhage in advanced cases. Despite adrenal haemorrhage, the adrenal medulla more than cortex is destroyed, and these patients do not have low plasma cortisol levels. Giving steroids may worsen, not improve, the prognosis.

Management

Sulphonamides were very effective, but sulphonamide-resistant meningococci have now spread worldwide, and treatment should be with benzylpenicillin (penicillin G) or amoxycillin.

1. Benzylpenicillin, 2×10^6 units 4-hourly or amoxycillin 1–2 g 4-hourly by small bolus i.v. infusion for 7 days. The pulse injection of penicillin should be slow, to avoid induction of ventricular tachyarrhythmias.

2. If the first lumbar puncture fluid is purulent, and clinical presentation not typical of meningococcal meningitis, 5000–20 000 units intrathecal penicillin may be given, the dose dependent on the age of the patient. The total daily dose of benzylpenicillin should not exceed 24×10^6 units because of possible encephalopathy, although this is very rare below 48×10^6 units daily.

3. In the penicillin-allergic patient, chloramphenicol, 2–4 g daily (1 g 6-hourly), should be given for at least 5 days in adults, 100 mg/kg in children, half this dose in neonates.

4. If the patient has thrombocytopenia or DIC, intravenous antibiotic therapy is mandatory, but in other patients the intramuscular route may be used after 2 days.

5. For the patient in agony with headache, diamorphine or pethidine can be given, and nausea prevented by domperidone.

6. In fulminant septicaemia with shock, hydrocortisone hemisuccinate 200 mg i.v. has been given, but this is contentious, since steroids may impair the patient's response to acute infection, and fluid and electrolyte balance.

7. In the early stages of a consumption coagulopathy (see p. 39), bolus injections of heparin 10 000–15 000 units should be given, as this may prevent thrombosis, but further heparin can cause bleeding.

8. Seizures may be due to meningitis, but also to neurotoxicity from massive doses of penicillin, or from electrolyte disturbances, in particular hyponatraemia. A loading dose of phenytoin (see p. 64) should be given, with diazepam if status epilepticus is present.

9. If there are signs of cerebral oedema with tentorial or cerebellar herniation, mannitol 20% i.v. has a rapid action. With appropriate treatment, mortality from acute meningococcal meningitis in otherwise healthy young adults is approximately 5%–10%.

Hemophilus influenzae Meningitis

In Britain, *H. influenzae* meningitis is largely confined to children under 3 years, but it is a common cause of meningitis in adults in other countries. The disease has a 10%–15% mortality. The drug of choice is chloramphenicol in the following dosage: neonates, 50 mg/kg daily; children, 100 mg/kg daily; adults, 4 g daily. Chloramphenicol should be given 6-hourly i.v., although it can subsequently be given p.o., and diffuses well into the cerebrospinal fluid.

Ampicillin, 75–200 mg/kg daily, or preferably amoxycillin, is an alternative to chloramphenicol. High doses are necessary to achieve adequate CSF concentration. There have been cases of chloramphenicol (and of ampicillin) resistance, usually responsive to cefotaxime (see p. 114).

Treatment should continue for 5–10 days, depending on clinical response. In some instances, persistent fever abates when antibacterial drugs are stopped. The level of consciousness may remain impaired for a few days following cerebrospinal fluid sterilisation, although other causes of impaired consciousness should be sought.

Pneumococcal Meningitis

Pneumococcal meningitis mostly affects young infants or the elderly in Britain, where it is the commonest form of meningitis, with a mortality as high as 50%. Predisposing causes (see p. 100), sinus infection, skull fracture, alcoholism and immunological dysfunction, must be sought. The prodromal illness is often less acute than in meningococcal meningitis, and a rash is unusual. The condition is diagnosed by the finding of pneumococci in the Gram-stained purulent CSF. The treatment of choice is with i.v. amoxycillin, as for meningococcal meningitis, with initial intrathecal dosage; or perhaps more satisfactorily with cephalosporins (see p. 113).

In pneumococcal meningitis, treatment should continue for 14 days after the fever has remitted, and for at least 3 weeks in infections with Gram-negative organisms, since the relapse rate is high in these cases.

Neonatal Meningitis

Bacterial meningitis appears in the first month of life more frequently than at any other time. It is especially common in premature infants, and in neonates with spina bifida. Many of these infections are caused by Gram-negative organisms, particularly *Escherichia coli*, *Proteus* spp. and *Pseudomonas aeruginosa*, but are also sometimes due to listeria, streptococci and staphylococci. Intrathecal and intraventricular gentamicin 1 mg/day combined with parenteral gentamicin 4–8 mg kg^{-1} day^{-1}, continued for 10–14 days, is effective for most of these Gram-negative organisms. Prolonged fever, fits and subdural effusions may arise during treatment, and some paediatricians use daily intrathecal corticosteroids.

Recurrent Bacterial Meningitis

This is usually caused by pneumococci, in patients with skull defects, especially fractures of the anterior fossa across the cribriform plate, but also occasionally following splenectomy or with lymphoreticular disease. These patients must be carefully investigated for CSF leak or fistula, with surgical closure when found. Patients with CSF rhinorrhoea or otorrhoea are at risk of meningitis, and should be treated prophylactically with penicillin V, 500 mg four times daily p.o. until the leak stops.

Rare Forms of Meningitis

Fungal

Infection with *Cryptococcus neoformans* is rare, and about half the patients have altered immunity, diabetes mellitus or sarcoidosis, although some patients are apparently otherwise healthy. *C. neoformans* may cause meningitis, encephalitis or an expanding focal lesion.

Aspergillosis usually affects immunocompromised or renal transplant patients. Neurological symptoms usually begin suddenly with stroke-like deficits associated with vessel invasion, mycotic aneurysms or multiple cerebral abscesses, in the hemispheres, brain stem and cerebellum, with focal areas of meningitis. Bronchoscopy, and/or cerebral biopsy, may be necessary to make the diagnosis. Although amphotericin B will cure pulmonary aspergillosis, aspergillosis of the nervous system has a high mortality, despite treatment.

Amphotericin B and flucytosine (see p. 120) have improved prognosis in these previously invariably fatal conditions, but adverse effects are common. Recent alternatives (miconazole, or the imidazole antifungal drug ketoconazole) appear to be no more effective than amphotericin.

Protozoa

Toxoplasmosis as a cause of meningoencephalitis is most common in laboratory workers exposed to virulent strains or in immunocompromised patients, whilst generalised infection by *Toxoplasma gondii* arises most commonly by crossing the placenta. Treatment should be started with pyrimethamine 0.5 mg kg^{-1} day^{-1} combined with sulphadimidine 3 g daily. This may result in neutropenia or thrombocytopenia, in which case spiramycin 2 mg daily should be used.

Bacteria

Legionellosis, although first described and usually presenting with pneumonia, involves many other organs, and the central and peripheral nervous systems are involved in most patients, with focal neurological signs and sometimes a peripheral neuritis. Nervous system damage appears to be due to an endotoxin rather than direct bacterial infection.

Listeria monocytogenes meningitis or brain abscess is most common in the elderly and the immunosuppressed, but sometimes arises in pregnancy or in apparently healthy adults. Amoxycillin, 100 mg kg^{-1} day^{-1}, in divided doses, or chloramphenicol, is generally effective.

Streptococcal meningitis is very uncommon, except following head injury or cranial surgery. Benzylpenicillin should be given intrathecally and by 4-h pulse intravenous injection. Staphylococcal meningitis is usually associated with a mucky shunt, fulminating bacteraemia, or is seen after head trauma. Parenteral cephaloridine or methicillin should be given.

In adults, Gram-negative bacterial meningitis due to *E. coli*, *Proteus* spp., *Pseudomonas aeruginosa*, or *Aerobacter aerogenes*, is associated with head trauma, surgery or systemic disease. Many of these patients are severely ill or refractory to many antibiotics; and the prognosis is generally poor. Gentamicin systemically, intrathecally or intraventricularly, via an implanted reservoir, amoxycillin, carbenicillin, cefotaxime or chloramphenicol systemically, should be given, and may occasionally save the patient.

Brain Abscess

Brain abscesses are almost invariably secondary to pus elsewhere in the body; the nasal sinuses, middle ear, mastoid air cells, sepsis in the lungs, or infected heart valves. In 10%–20% of cases, no source can be found. Subacute bacterial endocarditis rarely if ever gives rise to brain abscess, but acute bacterial endocarditis due to virulent staphylococci or other pathogens may produce multiple small infected cerebral lesions.

The most common organisms found in brain abscesses are anaerobic streptococci, often originating in the lung or in infected nasal sinuses. Post-traumatic and spinal abscesses are usually caused by *Staphylcoccus aureus*. Ear infections leading to cerebral abscess are often associated with enteric organisms.

Surgical treatment during the stage of acute cerebral abscess formation usually accomplishes little, and excision is impossible until the abscess has become clearly localised with a definite wall. On the other hand, antibiotics do not penetrate abscesses well, but even without bacteriological examination of the intracerebral mass, certain antibiotics can be used, starting treatment empirically with benzylpenicillin 24×10^6 units, and chloramphenicol 4 g daily, i.v. in divided doses. Metronidazole is of value in the treatment of enteric-derived bacterial abscesses associated with middle ear infection.

Neurosyphilis

The risk of neurosyphilis following treated primary or secondary syphilis is difficult to determine, perhaps 5%–10%. The aim of treatment for syphilis must be to prevent tertiary disease, before any major damage to the heart, blood vessels or central nervous system has occurred.

Untreated tertiary syphilis is very uncommon in the United Kingdom, although positive syphilis serology occurs in 1%–2% of all patients attending a general neurology outpatient clinic, particularly in subjects from areas of the world in which yaws, pinta or bejel are endemic. The clinical diagnosis of neurosyphilis can be difficult unless classic signs of taboparesis are present, and the usual problem is how to treat a variety of minor neurological complaints such as headache, unsteadiness, or root pain, or more major problems including deafness, visual problems, and uveitis, in a patient with positive serology. The management of these patients presents considerable difficulties. Yaws, pinta and bejel are nonvenereal diseases produced by treponemes which are antigenically similar to *Treponema pallidum*, but which produce distinct skin, bone or mucous membrane lesions. The most specific routine test for syphilis, the fluorescent treponemal absorption (FTA) antibody test, shows cross-reactivity between antibodies for *T. pallidum* and *T. pertenue*. In the absence of any test that will distinguish between the two treponemes, it is wise to assume the presence of the more serious infection. The nonvenereal treponemes are sometimes considered to produce central nervous system involvement, but in the absence of antigenic specificity this cannot be proven.

If the patient will submit to investigation, and the cerebrospinal fluid proves to be entirely normal, then neurosyphilis can be safely excluded. However, in other circumstances, when the FTA is positive but lumbar puncture refused, a syphilitic aetiology should be considered for any undiagnosed neurological illness, with the possible exception of parkinsonism and a pure cerebellar syndrome; and the patient should be treated for treponemal infection. Treatment is similar for all the treponematoses.

The next problem is to decide what is adequate treatment for neurosyphilis. This is still unknown, since progression may occur despite massive doses of antibiotics. Some experts have considered that intravenous benzylpenicillin, in doses as high as $18–24 \times 10^6$ units daily given for 10 days, is necessary if any immune marker is present in the CSF. The current recommendation is for at least 6×10^6 units penicillin, and at least double this quantity is usually given (e.g. benzathine benzylpenicillin G 2.4×10^6 units i.m. weekly for 4 weeks; or procaine penicillin 1.2 g daily for at least 10 days, usually combined with probenecid 500 mg twice daily). If neither regime is successful, and symptoms progress, a course of high-dose intravenous penicillin must be given, combined with high-dose prednisolone (80 mg daily). Few physicians today are familiar with the Jarisch–Herxheimer reaction, an acute febrile response due to the liberation of huge quantities of treponemal antigen; this can probably be avoided by combining penicillin with a high dose of prednisolone for the first 3 days of treatment. Prednisolone 80 mg daily should also be given to patients with syphilitic inner ear disease, or with uveitis, until symptoms are reversed. Unfortunately, there is no clear evidence that steroid treatment will prevent the occasional progression of optic atrophy attributed to syphilis.

Tuberculous Meningitis

Tuberculous meningitis is now comparatively uncommon in the United Kingdom. It is seen most often in childhood or in early adult life, but also occurs in the elderly. The diagnosis is often missed. If there is a chronic meningitis, despite normal CSF findings and no evidence of tuberculosis on Ziehl–Neelsen staining, with no other organisms present, antituberculous treatment should be considered.

After the introduction of each new antituberculous drug there has been a decrease in tuberculosis mortality. Experience with these modern drugs has been greatest in the less developed countries, and suggests that initial four-drug treatment gives the best results, using isoniazid, rifampicin, ethambutol and pyrazinamide. The addition of pyrazinamide to the other drugs results in a considerable increase in overall bactericidal effect, and the total duration of necessary therapy is shortened.

After the initial 12 weeks' treatment, and when sensitivities are known, four-drug treatment may be replaced by two-drug therapy (e.g. isoniazid and rifampicin daily for 6 months; longer if pyrazinamide has not been included in initial treatment). Drug toxicity with all these regimes is fairly high.

1. Isoniazid must be combined with pyridoxine, 50–100 mg daily, to prevent vitamin depletion and subsequent neuropathy, myelopathy or, rarely, encephalopathy.

2. Rifampacin may cause liver damage, which is usually reversible. In 20%–30% of subjects, other toxicity symptoms, influenzal, respiratory or abdominal symptoms, shock, renal failure or purpura, occur.

3. Ethambutol may cause initial subjective defects in vision, followed by loss of visual acuity, colour blindness, and restriction in visual fields. Initially these changes are dose-related, and are reversed on stopping the drug. However, ethambutol should not be given to patients in whom careful visual monitoring is impossible.

4. Pyrazinamide is hepatotoxic, and may cause jaundice, anorexia, hepatomegaly, nausea and vomiting, as well as arthralgia, sideroblastic anaemia and urticaria.

With these regimes, a success rate of 80%–90% can be obtained in tuberculous meningitis when treatment is supervised and drug intake is regular. The total treatment period should be not less than 9 months, and patients should remain under surveillance for at least 12 months after treatment is stopped. Effective chemotherapy has largely abolished the need for immobilisation in spinal tuberculosis.

The use of steroids in meningeal tuberculosis is controversial. Some experts give corticosteroids to all cases of tuberculous meningitis for at least the first week of treatment, and corticosteroids are life-saving in patients who develop cerebral oedema, possibly an allergic reaction to tuberculin after treatment starts. There is no doubt that steroids help the resolution of overwhelming pulmonary infection at the commencement of antituberculous therapy, and they should probably also be used in all drug-resistant meningeal cases with progressive disease or tuberculoma formation.

Viral Meningoencephalitis

Viral meningitis is common and, with the exception of mumps, is largely due to small RNA enteroviruses, including Coxsackie, echoviruses and polio. No specific treatment is available for most of these illnesses but, with the exception of poliomyelitis, the condition is usually benign, except in the rare case of agammaglobulinaemia, or in the presence of immune suppression. Many of these diseases are most common in late summer, and are spread by contact with infected individuals in the presence of poor sanitation. In contrast, meningoencephalitis following influenza, measles, mumps and rubella is mainly a disease of the winter months.

Meningoencephalitis due to DNA viruses is less common than following RNA virus infection. Chickenpox, caused by the DNA varicella zoster virus, results in meningoencephalitis in 1 in 2000 cases. Shingles (herpes zoster) is probably due to reactivation of dormant virus in trigeminal or dorsal root ganglia. Herpes simplex virus (types 1 and 2) is a common orogenital DNA virus which occasionally causes severe meningoencephalitis. Herpes simplex virus type 2 infection of the nervous system is mainly restricted to newborn infants who may acquire infection via an infected maternal genital tract. Epstein–Barr virus, associated with most cases of infectious mononucleosis, causes many different neurological sequelae, although meningoencephalitis is rare.

Specific treatment for RNA virus infection of the nervous system has not been achieved. Treatment of DNA herpes virus infection with acyclovir is, however, effective. There is still no effective treatment for subacute sclerosing panencephalitis (SSPE), slow virus infection of animals, or Jakob–Creutzfeldt disease in humans.

Amantadine, first synthesised in the Du Pont laboratories, has some anti-influenzal (RNA virus) action, attributed to inhibition of viral enzymes and the prevention of viral uncoating on cellular entry, but is not effective against the common RNA viruses that attack the nervous system, or against DNA virus infection.

Amantadine hydrochloride 100–200 mg daily has been investigated in SSPE and Jakob–Creutzfeldt disease. There are six isolated reports that amantadine causes improvement in the clinical state and EEG in early cases of Jakob–Creutzfeldt disease. However, improvement is at best slight or temporary, and may be due, not to any specific antiviral effect, but to the alerting action of this drug. Amantadine is not effective in animal scrapie.

Amantadine has a slight in vitro inhibitory effect on measles virus, but is almost certainly ineffective in SSPE, although Robertson et al. (1980) found sustained improvement in 4 of 38 children with SSPE treated with amantadine at the University of Kentucky, Lexington, between 1965 and 1978. The natural history of SSPE is very variable, and a few untreated patients have very substantial remissions lasting months or years.

Herpes Simplex Infection of the Nervous System

Herpes virus infection may account for some cases of benign recurrent aseptic meningitis (Mollaret's meningitis), with repeated attacks of meningism, CSF pleocytosis, fever and myalgia. Herpes simplex type 1 virus, shown by EM studies or by immunofluorescence, has been isolated from patients during an attack. Acyclovir (see p. 121) should be given. Herpes simplex also causes a severe fulminant necrotising encephalitis, as well as ocular disease.

Before the introduction of acyclovir, a great deal of effort was devoted to the laboratory diagnosis of herpes simplex encephalitis, using brain biopsy or blood and cerebrospinal fluid antibody detection of herpes virus antigen, since the then available treatment with cytosine arabinoside gave poor results and was very toxic (see, e.g. Klapper et al. 1981).

Acyclovir (acycloguanosine) is many times more effective than cytosine arabinoside or adenine arabinoside, as well as much less toxic. It has been shown to have great specificity for the herpes virus group in numerous clinical trials in both immunosuppressed and nonimmunosuppressed patients. It is administered by infusion over 1 h (repeated over 8 h), although oral preparations are now being tested. The drug is widely distributed throughout the body, with CSF levels approximately half those of plasma levels. Toxicity is minimal, although the solution for injection is somewhat irritant, with a pH of 10–11.

The availability, low toxicity and effectiveness of acyclovir have made the problem of brain biopsy in suspected herpes simplex infections redundant. It is better to go ahead anyway and treat early if the condition is suspected on clinical grounds, even if the results of CSF plasma studies are not available or even sometimes negative.

Topical acyclovir will control keratoconjunctivitis induced by herpes zoster as well as herpes simplex ocular disease. In herpes zoster ophthalmicus, treated with acyclovir, ocular herpes quickly resolves, sometimes in 5–6 days. Not all patients respond, however, to low-dosage oral or intravenous acyclovir, and high dosage (800 mg daily p.o.) may be necessary to treat herpes zoster ophthalmicus.

If necessary, acyclovir may be combined with steroids to suppress uveitis with ocular herpes, although this may cause delayed resolution, and the intravenous infusion is used in the treatment of herpes simplex infections (acyclovir 5 mg/kg by slow i.v. infusion). It has not yet been convincingly shown whether acyclovir will prevent postherpetic neuralgia.

The efficacy of acyclovir for other neurological complications of herpes zoster has not been investigated in detail but, in zoster myelitis, acyclovir 800 mg daily is sometimes dramatically successful, as is also the case in disseminated zoster, with bone marrow suppression or renal insufficiency. Epstein–Barr virus is sensitive in vitro to acyclovir, and there is a potential role for the treatment of neurological disorders in infectious mononucleosis.

Trials of other antiviral drugs, interferons, phosphonoformate in cutaneous herpes, and deoxyuridine derivatives, are currently under way. The number of effective antiviral drugs, at least for DNA viruses, is likely to increase greatly during the next decade.

Reye's Syndrome

Reye's syndrome, a viral illness followed by repeated vomiting, signs of hepatic encephalopathy, delirium, coma and seizures, with a very high blood ammonia level, as well as increase in free fatty acids, is a toxic or metabolic disorder. At present Reye's syndrome is the second most common cause of death from virus-associated diseases with CNS involvement in the paediatric age group. It may result from hepatic mitochondrial dysfunction. Pathologically, fatty changes in the liver and diffuse cerebral oedema are observed. The condition is largely confined to children, and is much less common in adolescents and young adults. Several thousand patients have been described. Early figures suggested a very high mortality, perhaps 60%–80% but, with increasing recognition of mild cases and more effective treatment, survival in many children and a few adults has now been reported.

In Reye's syndrome, exchange transfusion and peritoneal dialysis give no benefit over other methods of treatment. The combination of neomycin enemas to reduce hyperammonaemia, intravenous hypertonic glucose to prevent hypoglycaemia, insulin to prevent further fatty acid release, cooling in the presence of severe hyperthermia, as well as reduction of often strikingly elevated cerebrospinal fluid pressure with steroids, controlled ventilation and, if necessary, mannitol, results in a marked reduction in mortality. In a series of children with Reye's syndrome reported by Trauner (1980) treated by these methods, all survived. Recently it has been suggested that the use of salicylates during an antecedent viral illness may be associated with Reye's syndrome.

Antibiotic Pharmacology

Penicillins

The penicillins fall into three main groups:

1. Benzylpenicillin (which is highly soluble, but unstable at acid pH) and alternatives to it that are resistant to gastric acid.

2. Penicillinase-resistant penicillins (e.g. methicillin, cloxacillin), which are used only against penicillinase-producing staphylococci.

3. Broad-spectrum penicillins such as ampicillin and amoxycillin, which are not penicillinase-resistant.

The penicillins have a bactericidal action. They block the production of glycopeptide cross-linkages used in the formation of bacterial cell walls. The affected cell walls lack normal rigidity and are destroyed by osmotic forces. Since existing bacterial cell walls are not damaged, bacteria must be in a state of growth or multiplication in order to be destroyed by penicillins, which should therefore not be given with bacteriostatic antibiotics. They can act synergistically with other bactericidal antibiotics.

Benzylpenicillin acts mainly on Gram-positive organisms, principally streptococci, penicillinase-negative staphylococci, clostridia, *Bacillus anthracis*, corynebacteria, and *Listeria monocytogenes*. Benzylpenicillin is also active against certain Gram-negative organisms, notably *Neisseria meningitidis*, *Neisseria gonorrhoeae* (sometimes resistant) and *Treponema pallidum*. It is also active against actinomyces.

Cloxacillin is resistant to penicillinase, and is used solely against penicillinase-producing staphylococci, since its activity is otherwise less than that of benzylpenicillin.

Ampicillin (adult dose in meningitis 12–24 g/day i.v. in six divided doses) is a broad-spectrum antibiotic, not resistant to penicillinase and less active against most Gram-positive organisms than benzylpenicillin. It is usually active against *Hemophilus influenzae*, salmonellae, shigellae and some *Escherichia coli*, proteus and klebsiella strains. Amoxycillin has a similar spectrum, and is rather better absorbed orally. Ampicillin is overall nontoxic, but does cause occasional hypersensitivity reactions—not an indication to stop therapy—and, very rarely, encephalopathy and seizures.

Carbenicillin is mainly used against pseudomonas and some proteus and serratia.

Oral benzylpenicillin is largely destroyed by gastric acid, but 10%–30% may be absorbed, mainly from the duodenum, with t_{max} 0.5–1 h. Phenoxymethylpenicillin, which is acid-resistant, is less active against some important pathogens. Carbenicillin too is not acid-stable, and when given i.m., peak levels are reached in about 1 h. In serious infections when penicillin is indicated, benzylpenicillin is given parenterally. When given intramuscularly, peak levels of benzylpenicillin are reached in about 0.5 h. Cloxacillin is acid-stable and 30%–50% bioavailable when given by mouth. Ampicillin is acid-stable, and well absorbed on oral administration. Peak plasma level is at 2 h. When given intramuscularly, peak level is reached in 1 h.

The penicillins have good penetration to most tissues, but poor entry to CSF. In treating meningitis, this is compensated for by giving large doses intravenously. Cloxacillin is strongly (95%) bound to plasma proteins, the others less strongly. Ampicillin reaches 10%–50% of blood level in the CSF, but benzylpenicillin hardly penetrates to CSF (1%–6% of blood level), and carbenicillin not at all. Penetration of antibiotics into the CSF is increased when the meninges are inflamed, and this is usually attributed to impairment of the blood–brain barrier. However, it has also been suggested that some antibiotics are actively excreted from CSF by choroid plexus, by a mechanism which extrudes organic acids from CSF, which is blocked by probenecid, and which is disabled in meningitis. Penetration of penicillins into cerebral abscesses is slow and poor, so that very high plasma levels are needed to attain a bactericidal level in the abscess.

Penicillins are excreted mainly unchanged in the urine (Table 6.2), both by glomerular filtration and by active transport in the proximal tubule. Probenecid blocks tubular transport of penicillins, and loss by glomerular filtration is reduced in renal failure. Penicillins are not known to be metabolised by the liver, and the breakdown of penicillins by penicillinase-producing bacteria does not account for a significant proportion of a dose, or accelerate the fall in blood levels following a dose. The half-lives of penicillins vary from 0.5 to 1.5 h, but 6-hourly dosage can maintain a bactericidal level to sensitive organisms, as the peak level is many times the minimal lethal concentration.

Penicillin hypersensitivity can be manifested by urticarial skin rash or pruritus. A subsequent dose can then cause an anaphylactic reaction, and even death. Haemolytic anaemia or nephritis occurs rarely. Penicillin is a convulsant when it reaches the brain, so intrathecal dosage should not exceed 20 000 units in adults, and 3–10 000 units in children. Very high blood levels, achieved by very large dosage (or normal dosage in the presence of renal insufficiency) can lead to convulsant CSF penicillin levels, particularly in meningitis. Penicillins are given as their sodium or potassium salts, and in large dosage can cause electrolyte imbalance, again particularly in renal failure.

Cephalosporins

Cephalosporium acremonium elaborates three antibacterial compounds, of which one (cephalosporin C) is resistant to penicillinase and bactericidal to a wide range of pathogens, including common pathogens such as *E. coli*, *Klebsiella* spp., and *Proteus* spp. Cephalosporins are of great value in treating severe undiagnosed sepsis.

The cephalosporins act in a qualitatively and quantitatively similar way to the penicillins, which they resemble structurally. However, they are resistant to staphylococcal penicillinase, which binds to but does not inactivate them. Although cephalosporins act as competitive and noncompetitive inhibitors of penicillinase, they do not prevent the breakdown of penicillins concurrently given.

Cephalosporins combine penicillinase resistance with a broad spectrum rather similar to that of ampicillin. They are not reliably active against *N. meningitidis* or *N. gonorrhoeae*. Cephalosporins are active against a wide range of Gram-positive and Gram-negative organisms. Group A *Streptococcus pyogenes*, *Streoptococcus viridans*, nonhaemolytic streptococci, *Diplococ-*

Table 6.2. Pharmacokinetics of some antimicrobial drugs

Drug	Oral absorption		Distribution		Penetration into CSF	Elimination	
	Fraction (%)	t_{max} (h)	V_d (l/kg)	Binding (%)		$t_{1/2}$ (h)	Unchanged (%)
Benzylpenicillin	30 (good i.m.)	0.5–1	0.3	65	a	0.5	60–90
Ampicillin	50	2	0.39	23	Yes	1–1.5	90
Amoxycillin	100	2	0.3	25	Yes	5	60
Cloxacillin	30–50	0.5–1	0.35	95	Poor	0.4	78
Carbenicillin	5 (good i.m.)	0.5–1 (i.m.)	0.17	50	No	1	82
Cephaloridine	5 (good i.m.)	0.5 (i.m.)	0.3	20–35	a	0.5–1	60–90
Cephalothin	2 (good i.m.)	0.5 (i.m.)	0.26	50–80	Poor	5	60–90
Cephalexin	50–80	0.5–1	0.23	6–15	a	4–8	60–100
Cefotaxime	5 (good i.m.)	0.5 (i.m.)	0.8	40	a	1–1.5	60–80
Chloramphenicol	Good	2	0.57	25–60	Good	2–3	5–15
Gentamicin	5 (good i.m.)	1–2 (i.m.)	0.3	0	No	1–4	70–80
Streptomycin	0 (good i.m.)	1–2 (i.m.)	0.26	20–30	a	2.5–5	65
Rifampicin	Good	1–2	0.93	84–91	a	2.8–4	12
Isoniazid (fast)	Good	1–3	0.6	20–30	Good	1–1.25	65
Isoniazid (slow)	Good	1–3	0.6	50	Good	2.5–3.5	57–66
Ethambutol	75–80	4	1	40	Poor	4.2	70–80
Dapsone	100	4–6	1	50	Yes	18–48	70

a CSF penetration in presence of inflammation

cus pneumoniae, Staphylococcus aureus (penicillinase-positive and -negative), *Staphylococcus epidermidis, Clostridium welchii, L. monocytogenes, Bacillus subtilis, Corynebacterium diphtheriae, N. gonorrhoeae, N. meningitidis* and *Actinomyces israelii* are often sensitive at 0.004–1.0 μg/ml. Most salmonella, including *S. typhosa,* most shigella, all *Proteus mirabilis,* about 75% of *E. coli,* 60% of paracolons, and 50% of *H. influenzae,* are sensitive at 4–16 μg/ml. *Clostridium aerogenes* and *Pseudomonas aeruginosa* make a different β-lactamase which destroys cephalosporins (cephalosporinase).

Cephaloridine and the cephalothin class are poorly absorbed from the gut. They are rapidly absorbed intramuscularly and are widely distributed. Cephalexin and its congeners are acid-stable, and rapidly absorbed orally.

The cephalosporins are widely distributed in body water, but hardly enter CSF, except in meningeal inflammation, when the CSF level may reach 1% of plasma level. Cefotaxime is the exception, and its CSF level is high in meningeal inflammation, and often bactericidal, even with normal meninges. The apparent volume of distribution is larger than that of penicillins.

The cephalosporins are largely excreted unchanged in urine. The plasma half-life of cephaloridine is 50 min, of cephalothin and cephalexin about 2 h. Cephaloridine is excreted by glomerular filtration, cephalothin also by tubular secretion, so its excretion can be slowed with probenecid. About 25% of a dose of cephalothin is excreted in the urine as the *o*-deacetylated derivative. Cefotaxime is deacetylated to a somewhat less active metabolite, with a plasma half-life of about 2 h. Half-life in CSF is several times as long.

In about 5% of cases, a sensitivity reaction can occur to cephalosporins, with fever, urticaria, eosinophilia, morbilliform rashes and anaphylaxis. Most patients hypersensitive to penicillins are not sensitive to cephalosporins, but cross-sensitivity occurs in 10% of penicillin-sensitive patients. Cephaloridine (but not the others) can cause renal tubular necrosis, and high dosage usually results in many granular casts. For this reason, cephaloridine is no longer in general use.

Chloramphenicol

Chloramphenicol (adult dose in meningitis 4 g daily in four divided doses; infants over 2 months 50–100 mg kg^{-1} day^{-1}; under 2 months 25–50 mg kg^{-1} day^{-1}) is bacteriostatic in low concentration (8–10 μg/ml) against many Gram-negative organisms, such as *E. coli, Klebsiella pneumoniae, Bordetella pertussis, H. influenzae, Enterobacter aerogenes, Salmonella typhi, Vibrio cholerae,* pasteurella, bacteroides, and some strains of neisseria, shigella, and brucella. At moderate concentrations it is active against *B. anthracis, C. diphtheriae,* actinomyces, clostridia, listeria and leptospira, rickettsia, chlamydia and mycoplasma.

Chloramphenicol is well absorbed orally, with t_{max} about 2 h. Peak plasma level after a dose of 4 g is 20–40 μg/ml. It is distributed throughout body water. It rapidly penetrates into CSF, where its concentration reaches 10%–60% of that in plasma. It reaches bile and milk, and crosses the placenta. It is largely metabolised by conjugation to the glucuronide and hydrolysis in the urine. The unchanged drug is filtered, and the glucuronide secreted by the renal tubules.

Theoretically, chloramphenicol may interfere with the bactericidal action of penicillins. It can block the action of haematinics by inhibiting the uptake of iron into red cell precursors. Its antibacterial effect on gut flora can reduce synthesis of vitamin K in the gut, and so cause hypoprothrombinaemia. It may prolong the action of other drugs by inhibiting their biotransformation in the liver (e.g. tolbutamide, chlorpropamide, phenytoin). Occasionally rashes, angioneurotic oedema and fever occur.

The most serious toxic effect of chloramphenicol is bone marrow aplasia with pancytopenia, and this is often fatal. This rare, irreversible bone marrow suppression is idiosyncratic, not dose-related, but usually occurs only after prolonged or repeated treatment with chloramphenicol. For this reason, chloramphenicol is generally used only if no other drug will do. In contrast, dose-related bone marrow suppression due to iron uptake blockage in normoblasts is reversible, usually associated with plasma drug levels higher than 25 mg/ml. The earliest sign of this is increased serum iron and decreased reticulocyte count.

Nausea, vomiting, diarrhoea and perineal irritation occur, probably because of disturbance of normal gut flora. Peripheral and optic neuritis have been reported. Metabolism and excretion of chloramphenicol in neonates are poor, so that chloramphenicol can accumulate, resulting in a "grey baby syndrome", with vomiting, refusal to feed, abdominal distension and diarrhoea. Mortality is high.

Aminoglycosides

The aminoglycosides act in a number of ways on bacterial cells. They affect the integrity of the plasma membrane and the metabolism of RNA, but their most important action is on the bacterial ribosomes, with inhibition of protein biosynthesis. Streptomycin is an antibiotic which is bacteriostatic or bactericidal (depending on concentration) at 5–50 μg/ml plasma concentration against a number of Gram-negative organisms, but is widely used only in the treatment of tuberculosis.

Gentamicin (initial dose in meningitis in neonates 5 mg kg^{-1} day^{-1}; in infants 7.5 mg, i.v. or i.m.) is a mixture of antibiotic substances bactericidal at 5–10 μg/ml against many aerobic bacteria, such as *P. aeruginosa*, *E. coli*, klebsiella and enterobacter. Some strains of proteus are sensitive, as are many staphylococci, *H. influenzae*, bacteroides and *Mycobacterium tuberculosis*. It is active against streptococci.

When aminoglycosides are given i.m., the maximum blood level is reached in 1–2 h, with therapeutic levels persisting for 8–24 h. Serum blood levels should be monitored in meningitis. Streptomycin 1 g i.m. gives a peak plasma level of 20–30 μg/ml, and gentamicin 1 mg/kg, a peak plasma level of 3–5 μg/ml. Gentamicin levels over 5 μg/ml are likely to be ototoxic, and may also produce neuromuscular blockade and depression of renal function. Total dose should not exceed 50 g.

Distributed initially mainly to the extracellular space, aminoglycosides diffuse slowly into most body fluids except CSF. Even when meninges are inflamed, penetration through them is poor. Streptomycin can be given intrathecally mixed with CSF at not more than 5 mg/ml in a daily dose of up to 50 mg for adults. Gentamicin is given intrathecally up to 5 mg/day. Half-life of gentamicin in CSF is 5 h, and the level should not exceed 10 μg/ml. Streptomycin is 20%–30% protein-bound in plasma and gentamicin unbound. They are eliminated mainly or totally unchanged in the urine, with a plasma half-life of 2–3 h. No metabolites are known.

Idiosyncratic toxicity is not common for gentamicin, but streptomycin can cause skin rash or oedema, stomatitis, eosinophilia, fever, blood dyscrasias or anaphylactic shock. Both streptomycin and gentamicin are ototoxic, causing vertigo, tinnitus and sometimes deafness which may be permanent, particularly in older patients or in the presence of reduced renal function. Ototoxic effects are proportional to duration of treatment as well as blood level. Dihydrostreptomycin may be less toxic to the vestibular division, but more toxic to the auditory division. Aminoglycosides potentiate the effect of competitive neuromuscular blockers such as curare, and weaken patients with myasthenia. Excessive intrathecal dosage of gentamicin can cause seizures or respiratory arrest.

Antituberculous Drugs

Streptomycin

Streptomycin has already been considered.

Rifampicin

The rifamycins are a group of antibiotics obtained from *Streptomyces mediterranei*, and rifampicin is derived from rifamycin B. Rifampicin is bactericidal, and highly active against *M. tuberculosis*.

Rifamycins inhibit the growth of Gram-positive bacteria, including *M. tuberculosis* and penicillinase-producing staphylococci. Some Gram-negative organisms are sensitive, such as *N. meningitidis*, and some klebsiella, pseudomonas, proteus and *E. coli*. Therapeutic level for sensitive organisms is about 7 μg/ml. Rifampicin increases the antituberculous activity of streptomycin and isoniazid, but not of ethambutol. *M. tuberculosis* readily acquires resistance to rifampicin given alone.

Rifampicin is well absorbed orally, with peak plasma levels at 1–2 h. Rifampicin is largely (80%–90%) protein-bound in plasma, but it is distributed widely, and enters all body fluids including CSF, and crosses the placenta. A single dose of rifampicin 600 mg orally gives a peak plasma level of about 7 μg/ml. Elimination is largely by acetylation to an active metabolite which is secreted into bile and undergoes an enterohepatic circulation. Rifampicin induces hepatic acetylating enzymes, so its plasma half-life falls from an initial 4 h to about 2 h after 3 weeks, as well as accelerating the metabolism of other drugs. Both idiosyncratic and dose-related toxic effects can occur. Idiosyncratic leucopenia, purpura, thrombocytopenia and fever occur. Haematuria and renal failure have been reported. Dose-related effects include nausea, vomiting, diarrhoea, abdominal pain, lethargy, drowsiness, headache, dizziness, confusion, weakness and numbness. Liver toxicity occurs in slow acetylators, particularly if they are given isoniazid concurrently.

Isoniazid

Isoniazid is isonicotinic acid hydrazide, a polar and moderately soluble molecule. It is a potent antituberculous drug, cheap, and has a low toxicity. Isoniazid is active only against M. tuberculosis, in which it causes an accumulation of phosphorylated hexoses. It is not known whether this is the basis of its antibacterial effect. It is bacteriostatic or bactericidal, depending on concentration.

Isoniazid is well absorbed orally. Plasma levels should not exceed 1 μg/ml 24 h after the last dose. It is widely distributed throughout body water, and penetrates well into CSF, where its concentration is about 20% of that in plasma. Some 50% of plasma isoniazid is protein-bound.

Isoniazid is metabolised by acetylation, the rate of acetylation being bimodal and genetically determined, with the population divided into slow and fast acetylators. The plasma half-life is about 1 and 3 h for fast and slow acetylators, respectively. Slow acetylators therefore excrete about 60% of a dose unchanged in the urine, and fast acetylators only about 35%. About 60% of white people are slow acetylators, and adverse effects are confined mainly to this group. Dose-related toxicity in slow acetylators results in peripheral neuropathy, optic neuritis, myelopathy, epilepsy and encephalopathy. Neuropathy and perhaps the other neurological disturbances can be prevented with pyridoxine 50 mg daily, which should be given prophylactically to all slow acetylators given isoniazid, and all patients given high doses. Fever, skin rashes, hepatitis, vasculitis and bone marrow depression occur as an idiosyncratic reaction in both groups.

Ethambutol

A water-soluble secondary amine. The (+)-isomer is active. Ethambutol is a powerful bacteriostatic drug against many strains of M. tuberculosis, but not against other bacteria. Its mechanism of action is not known. Its antituberculous action is additive with that of streptomycin or isoniazid.

Resistance to ethambutol develops slowly if it is given alone. Ethambutol is well absorbed orally. About 75% of a dose is bioavailable. Peak plasma levels occur at about 2–4 h. One dose of ethambutol 25 mg/kg gives a peak plasma level of about 5 μg/ml, but it does not enter the CSF. Ethambutol is partly metabolised to an aldehyde and a dicarboxylic acid derivative; a variable amount is excreted unchanged in urine (15%–75%). Idiosyncratic toxic effects include skin rashes, joint pains, diarrhoea, fever, headache and confusion, and, rarely, anaphylaxis. An important dose-related toxic effect associated with dosages above 25 mg kg^{-1} day^{-1} is optic neuritis, only sometimes reversible. Plasma levels should be done, particularly in the presence of renal impairment or diabetes, as well as a regular ophthalmological assessment of visual acuity and colour vision.

Pyrazinamide

This nicotinic acid derivative penetrates the CSF well, and is a moderately potent bactericidal drug against *M. tuberculosis*. It is possibly more effective and certainly cheaper than ethambutol. Hepatotoxicity is the main risk, and serum transaminase levels should be estimated frequently during administration.

Antileprotic Drugs

Dapsone

Because of the worldwide importance of leprosy, dapsone is briefly considered here. Dapsone is one of a class of drugs (sulphones) which resemble sulphonamides and were synthesised during the flood of research that followed the discovery of the sulphonamides. Like the sulphonamides, the sulphones probably act by competitive block of uptake of *p*-aminobenzoic acid (PABA), and hence the synthesis of folic acid. Dapsone is bacteriostatic against *M. tuberculosis* as well as *M. leprae*, but is used mainly in the treatment of leprosy. Drug resistance in leprosy does occur, and dapsone may need to be combined with rifampicin, clofazimine or both. Dapsone is absorbed slowly but fairly completely when given orally, t_{max} being 1–3 h. It is widely distributed, and excreted in the bile with subsequent reabsorption and enterohepatic circulation. As a result of the enterohepatic circulation, dapsone has a plasma half-life of 18–48 h, and can be detected for up to 2 weeks. About 10% is excreted unchanged in the urine. Idiosyncratic toxic effects include anaemia, fever, haematuria and drug rashes. Anorexia, nausea, vomiting and a motor neuropathy occur as toxic effects, particularly in slow acetylators.

The lepra reaction can occur after several weeks of dapsone treatment of lepromatous leprosy, probably caused by sensitivity to released bacterial cell components, with erythematous nodules (erythema nodosum leprosum), fever, dermatitis, liver damage, lymphadenopathy and anaemia.

Antifungal Drugs

The three most widely used antifungal agents are amphotericin, griseofulvin and nystatin. Flucytosine is much less toxic than amphotericin, but it has a narrower spectrum, and its usefulness is limited by the development of resistance.

Amphotericin B is the current drug of choice for most systemic mycoses. It is a polyene fungicidal antibiotic produced by *Streptomyces nodosus*, and, closely resembling nystatin chemically, it is active against cryptococcus, candida and other yeasts, aspergillus, coccidioides and other fungi. It is amphoteric, and soluble in acid or alkaline solution (pH 2 or 11). Polyene antibiotics bind to sterol components of the membrane of sensitive fungi, increasing membrane permeability and leakage of intracellular components. Mammalian cell membranes contain similar sterols, so they are affected as well. The action of rifampicin is potentiated by amphotericin.

The main use of amphotericin in neurology is in the treatment of cryptococcal meningitis. It has also been suggested for use in amoebic encephalitis caused by free-living species such as *Acanthamoeba* spp. and *Naegleria* spp. It is used intrathecally and sometimes intraventricularly in meningitis due to *Cryptococcus* spp. or *Coccidioides immitis*.

Amphotericin can be used locally for superficial infections or by intravenous infusion for deep mycoses. Absorption by mouth is negligible. Treatment is started at 0.1–0.25 mg/kg infused daily, increasing slowly to 1–1.5 mg kg^{-1} day^{-1}, and followed by 0.6 mg/kg three times weekly up to a total of 2–3.5 g. About 10% is protein-bound. It does not enter the CSF, so it may need to be given intrathecally. Intrathecal amphotericin when given is diluted with CSF, starting with 0.025 mg/day and increasing to 0.5–1 mg/day. Amphotericin is eliminated slowly, with a plasma half-life of 1–2 days. A small proportion is secreted unchanged in urine.

Idiosyncratic toxic effects can occur, including anaphylaxis, thrombocytopenia, flushing, diffused pain and convulsions. Dose-related toxicity includes phlebitis, fever, headache, anorexia, anaemia, liver damage and jaundice, or kidney damage with consequent proteinuria, renal tubular acidosis, hypokalaemia and hypomagnesaemia. Intrathecal infusion can result in neuralgia, headache, paraesthesiae, foot drop, chemical meningitis and difficulty of micturition.

Flucytosine

Flucytosine (5-fluorocytosine) is a soluble pyrimidine analogue. It is converted by deamination into 5-fluorouracil, which is incorporated in the fungal tRNA, which may then be incapable of combining with the correct amino acids. Cytosine permease-deficient fungal mutants cannot take up cytosine or flucytosine, so they are unaffected by the drug. Flucytosine is inhibitory to *Cryptococcus neoformans, Aspergillus fumigatus, Sporotrichum schenckii* and some candida. Effective antifungal levels are usually in the range 5–12 µg/ml (oral dose 100–200 mg/kg daily in four divided doses).

Flucytosine is well absorbed orally, distributing to all body water. A single oral dose of 12–35 mg/kg gives peak plasma levels of about 30 µg/ml. This dose is given four times daily. About 50% of plasma level is protein-bound, and it penetrates CSF at 60%–90% of unbound plasma level. About 90% is excreted unchanged in urine, with a plasma half-life of 3–6 h. Combination of flucytosine with amphotericin allows a lower dose and shorter course of amphotericin to be given. Toxic effects are dose-related, and comprise nausea, vomiting, diarrhoea and skin rash, bone marrow depression, liver damage and jaundice, confusion, headaches, drowsiness and vertigo. Bone marrow suppression is the major problem, and is mainly avoided by drug level monitoring.

Antiviral Drugs

These are the least developed of antimicrobial drugs. They are mainly blockers of DNA synthesis, also used as antineoplastic and immunosuppressive agents. Their principal use in neurology is in the treatment of viral encephalitis, particularly herpes simplex encephalitis. Here, acyclovir has replaced other drugs.

Acyclovir

Used for the treatment of herpes simplex types 1 and 2, oral and genital infections, as well as herpes simplex encephalitis. It is less toxic than cytosine arabinoside and adenine arabinoside.

Acyclovir is phosphorylated to active triphosphate on entering the cell. It is about 20% bioavailable orally. Some is metabolised to 9-carboxymethoxymethylguanine. It is eliminated mainly unchanged in urine, both by glomerular filtration and tubular secretion. Plasma half-life with normal renal function is 3 h, in anuria 24 h.

Acyclovir acts as a substrate for, and inhibitor of, herpes-specific DNA polymerase, active against herpes simplex, types 1 and 2, and varicella zoster. For encephalitis it is usually given by i.v. infusion, for oral or genital herpes it is given p.o.

Idiosyncratic toxicity includes occasional rashes, liver impairment, bone marrow depression and neurological reactions. Significant dose-related effects are renal impairment (blood urea and creatinine elevation), and tissue damage and skin ulceration from accidental extravascular infusion.

Interferon

Very limited quantities of interferon have been available for trial in virus infection of the nervous system, eye, and herpes zoster. The therapeutic role of interferon in these conditions still has not been defined.

References

Klapper PE, Laing I, Longson M (1981) Rapid non-invasive diagnosis of herpes encephalitis. Lancet II: 607–609

Robertson WC Jr, Clark DB, Markesbery WR (1980) Review of 38 cases of subacute sclerosing panencephalitis: effect of amantadine on the natural course of the disease. Ann Neurol 8: 422–425

Trauner DA (1980) Treatment of Reye Syndrome. Ann Neurol 7: 2–4

7 Disorders of Sleep and Wakefulness

Daytime Drowsiness

Narcolepsy

Narcolepsy and sleep apnoea are the commonest causes of persistent daytime sleepiness. There are approximately 20 000 people with narcolepsy in the United Kingdom, 100 000 in the United States. The diagnosis of narcoleptic syndrome is established by the history of recurrent daily short sleep attacks in combination with cataplexy, brief episodes of loss of muscle tone and paralysis. Narcolepsy often results from monotony, and cataplexy is usually due to a sudden increase in alertness, with laughter or surprise. About one-half of all subjects also have sleep paralysis, and many describe vivid dreams at sleep onset, or even during wakefulness. In classic cases, the diagnosis is obvious from the history, and also from the finding of at least two sleep-onset REM periods during a multiple sleep latency test (MSLT). The MSLT gives an index of daytime drowsiness, with measurement of the time of sleep onset at 2-h intervals on five occasions throughout the day.

Many cases of narcolepsy are not classic in presentation, and the diagnosis is often missed for many years. All the clinical features may not be present, symptoms are sometimes poorly defined at the onset of the illness, and MSLT does not always show REM sleep onset. A diagnosis of the cause of daytime drowsiness sometimes cannot be firmly established in patients with brief sleep attacks alone, who have NREM sleep onset. The severity of daytime drowsiness in subjects with so-called monosymptomatic narcolepsy (i.e. narcolepsy with REM sleep onset, but no cataplexy or sleep paralysis) often warrants treatment.

Narcolepsy requires accurate diagnosis, and then usually lifelong treatment, since the condition does not remit. The recent discovery that all narcoleptics are HLA DR2-positive, as compared with only 20% of the normal population, may be helpful in diagnosis, since the finding of different D-related antigens probably excludes the diagnosis. Narcolepsy and cataplexy require separate treatment, and no one drug will abolish both symptoms.

The choice of drug for narcolepsy depends on the availability of effective CNS stimulants in different countries. Although narcoleptics do not usually abuse their treatment, amphetamine misuse by non-narcoleptic drug addicts has resulted in restricted availability of this class of compounds in many countries. However, there are at present no satisfactory alternatives to amphetamine and related drugs for the treatment of narcolepsy. Non-amphetamine derivatives which are sometimes recommended, including methysergide, monoamine oxidase A inhibitors, propranolol and nocturnal γ-hydroxybutyrate, are usually not very successful. Work regularity, planned short day sleep periods, and avoidance of monotony, all help to control narcolepsy.

Suggested choice of drugs for the treatment of narcolepsy is shown in Table 7.1. There is considerable individual response variation. With all these drugs, high dosages should be avoided if possible, but a very few severely disabled subjects require these, e.g. dexamphetamine 150 mg daily. This is usually due to rapid tolerance, a problem in about one-third of all narcoleptics given amphetamine. A drug holiday for 7–10 days may restore the initial effect in patients who complain of rapid loss of initial drug effectiveness over a few weeks. A sleep diary, kept by the patient, is often useful to monitor progress.

Table 7.1. Treatment for narcolepsy

Drug	Daily dose p.o. (mg)	Duration of stimulant effect of single dose (h)	Main advantages and problems
Mazindol	2–8	4–6	Little tolerance No effect on mood Not very potent Occasional gastro-intestinal irritation
Dexamphetamine	5–30 (doses higher than 60 mg daily have little or no additional stimulant effect)	Excretion is urinary pH-dependent; average 3–5	Tolerance in one-third of subjects Irritability and sweating are common
Fencamfamin	10–60	Slightly more prolonged effect than dexamphetamine	As dexamphetamine Tolerance common
Methylphenidate	10–60	3–5	May have different therapeutic ratio from dexamphetamine and preferred by some subjects Not generally available in the United Kingdom for new patients

Sympathomimetic side effects of central stimulant drugs are rarely a problem in the treatment of narcolepsy, although sweating, talkativeness, euphoria or mildly aggressive behaviour are not uncommon, in which case the dose of amphetamine should be reduced. Amphetamine given in the long term to narcoleptics does not produce serious anorexia or weight loss. Serious toxic effects, angiitis, myocardial infarction and amphetamine psychosis, are mainly if not entirely confined to drug addicts taking very large amphetamine doses.

Driving and Daytime Drowsiness

Severe daytime drowsiness is an important medical cause of road traffic accidents, although exact figures for the contribution of sleep apnoea and narcolepsy to road deaths are not available. Any serious degree of daytime drowsiness, whatever the cause, should result in driving disqualification. The problem of course is to define "serious", as well as allow for the effect of treatment. The MSLT may be useful under these circumstances.

Cataplexy

Clomipramine 10–150 mg p.o., given as a single evening dose, markedly reduces the frequency of cataplexy in about 80% of subjects. Other tricyclic drugs, imipramine and desmethylimipramine, are less effective than clomipramine. The anticataplectic effect of clomipramine, unlike the antidepressant effect, is immediate in onset. Drug withdrawal results in a severe rebound of cataplexy, which may last 3–4 days. Tolerance to clomipramine control of narcolepsy is less common than to amphetamine control of narcolepsy, although both occur.

Clomipramine–amphetamine combinations may theoretically cause hypertension, but this is not of practical importance in the treatment of narcolepsy–cataplexy; nor is the pharmacological finding that the stimulant effect of amphetamine may be enhanced somewhat by combination with tricyclic drugs.

Long-term clomipramine treatment of cataplexy results in an increase of appetite and weight gain in many subjects, as well as delayed ejaculation in males. Dosage of clomipramine, therefore, should be kept as low as possible, and alternate-day treatment is sometimes successful.

Idiopathic Hypersomnia

Daytime drowsiness can result from a large number of organic and psychiatric disorders, and an accurate diagnosis of these conditions is sometimes impossible. However, persistent day sleep attacks over many years, without cataplexy, drug or alcohol abuse, and with no evidence of any cerebral lesion, metabolic disease or respiratory disturbance, sleeping or waking, are usually due to one of three causes.

Monosymptomatic Narcolepsy

These subjects may have an affected relative, with all the clinical features of the narcoleptic syndrome, and also sleep-onset REM activity. Occasionally, the diagnosis of the narcoleptic syndrome is confirmed by the development of cataplexy—a gap of 40 years between the onset of narcolepsy and of cataplexy has been recorded. Treatment in these cases is with central stimulant drugs.

Endogenous Depression

A minority of patients with endogenous depression complain of hypersomnia, not insomnia, although otherwise the clinical features of depressive illness, which is not usually severe, are typical. The correct treatment for hypersomnia in these subjects is an antidepressant drug, and stimulant monoamine oxidase inhibitors are sometimes very successful.

Essential Hypersomnia

This condition is poorly defined, and the diagnostic status is unknown. The condition is characterised by excessive sleep throughout 24 h by day and night, with daytime drowsiness, frequent automatic behaviour, morning sleep drunkenness, and prolonged (over 10–12 h) and deep night sleep. Detailed neurological and psychiatric examination is necessary for diagnosis, and also polysomnogram studies, mainly to exclude sleep apnoea. Essential hypersomnolence may be lifelong, and is sometimes familial.

Pre-night-sleep-onset, stimulant drug treatment with ephedrine 30 mg, dexamphetamine 10 mg or mazindol 4 mg, may reduce the depth of night sleep, with subsequent improvement in daytime drowsiness. Alternatively, daytime stimulant drug treatment, as in narcolepsy, may be necessary.

Kleine–Levin Syndrome

The Kleine-Levin syndrome, periodic episodes of overeating with prolonged sleep and altered behaviour lasting a few days to 1–2 weeks, and recurring several times a year, is more common in males than females. The classic syndrome is uncommon, as most cases reported are atypical with, for example, a prominent psychiatric disturbance or no alteration in appetite. The condition is usually considered to be self-limiting, although this is not always so. The cause of the syndrome is completely unknown, and usually there is no disturbance of sleep, behaviour, appetite or sexual function between attacks. Some atypical examples have been associated with cyclical depression or the menarche.

Prophylaxis and treatment of the Kleine–Levin syndrome are both unsatisfactory. Lithium may prevent sleep episodes in cases associated with cyclical depression, and oestrogens occasionally improve menstrual-related hypersomnolence, even when normal ovulatory cycles are present. During an attack, amphetamines will alert sleepy patients, but often cause extreme irritability.

Parasomnias

The different parasomnias (literally events that happen around sleep) occur at different sleep stages and times at night (Table 7.2).

Table 7.2. The parasomnias

Stage of sleep	Parasomnia
Sleep onset	Hypnic jerks (normal)
	Bruxism, akathisia, sleep paralysis
First third of night)	Night terrors, somnambulism
(deep NREM sleep)	(enuresis—also during other sleep phases)
REM awakening	Nightmares, cluster headache, priapism
Last third of night	Asthma, cardiovascular disease, cardiac death

Most parasomnias are limited to childhood, and are worrying rather than serious. Treatment (Table 7.3) may require only parental reassurance. Psychiatric factors are of little or no importance, although sleepwalking, nocturnal enuresis and night terrors are worse at times of stress and following sleep loss. Behavioural therapy is usually not successful.

The commonest sleep problem in early childhood is difficulty in getting off to sleep, with marked restlessness. Behavioural management may be successful here, with the establishment of a restful environment, regular habits, and not paying too much attention to the sleepless child. Severe night hyperactivity and inability to sleep, sometimes in brain-damaged children, may require hypnotic or neuroleptic treatment.

Drug treatment of parasomnias is rarely of value. Children who sleepwalk may hurt themselves, and this should be guarded against. Disorders of arousal from deep stage 3–4 NREM sleep are alleviated by benzodiazepines (which reduce this sleep phase although this is unlikely to be the explanation for their effect). Long-term use in sedation is usually unacceptable in school-age children.

By far the most effective treatment for nocturnal enuresis is the buzzer and pad. Why this should work is uncertain, since arousal usually follows rather than precedes enuresis.

Table 7.3. Treatment of parasomnias

Parasomnia	Clinical features and differential diagnosis	Possible treatment
Sleep onset		
Hypnic jerks	Normal physiological event Distinguish from epilepsy	None needed
Sensory start	As hypnic jerk	None needed
Sleep paralysis	Familial; REM narcolepsy; or isolated Distinguish from periodic paralysis	Clomipramine 25 mg nocte
Hypnagogic hallucinations	Normal physiological event	
Bruxism	Usual age 2–15 or in elderly	Dental review; "bite guard"
Stage 3–4 NREM sleep (first third of night)		
Nocturnal enuresis	Up to 15% of normal children; more common in males Urological examination Not confined to NREM sleep	Ephedrine 15–30 mg Imipramine 10–25 mg Buzzer and pad
Sleepwalking	Up to 15% of normal children, but uncommon	Avoid injury Short-acting benzo-diazepine
Pavor nocturnus (night terror)	1%–4% of all children; males more than females Severe confusion; tachycardia; fear; screaming	As above; behavioural therapy may be of value
Middle and late sleep (REM sleep)		
Nightmares	Universal Good waking recall	None needed
Cluster headache (chronic paroxysmal hemicrania)	Wake patient Severe retro-orbital pain Sympathetic signs	Indomethacin Ergotamine
Nocturnal painful erection, priapism	Check Hb, clotting factors, blood pressure, vascular disease	Treat hypertension; suppress REM sleep (e.g. protriptyline)
Late night (mainly REM-sleep-related)		
Cardiovascular symptoms (e.g. angina) Gastro-oesophageal reflux	Distinguish from asthma, pharyngeal pouch, ulcer pain, etc.	Raise bed head
Abnormal swallowing		
Paroxysmal nocturnal haemoglobinuria during sleep	(Often chronic not paroxysmal): differentiate from haematuria, local genitourinary pathology, drug metabolites	Blood transfusion
Sleep myoclonus	Regular, rhythmic tibialis anterior jerks; usually occult May cause insomnia or daytime drowsiness Often associated with akathisia	Clonazepam 1–4 mg nocte[a] Cyproheptadine 4–8 mg nocte[a]
Sleep epilepsy	Usually generalised seizures or psychomotor attacks Peak occurrence first 2 h of sleep, with second peak at 4.00–5.00 a.m. Distinguish from night terrors and other automatisms	Anticonvulsants

[a] Treatment not of proven value.

Obstructive Sleep Apnoea

Obstructive sleep apnoea, due to anatomical narrowing and periodic collapse of the upper airway during sleep due to sleep atonia, is a common cause of daytime drowsiness. Most patients are male, overweight and over the age of 40, although obstructive sleep apnoea also occurs in children, sometimes associated with congenital mandibular-facial deformity.

The clinical diagnosis of obstructive sleep apnoea is established by a history of frequent, long (over 10 s, but sometimes as long as 90 s) apnoeas during sleep, ended with a loud explosive snort or honk as the airway resistance is overcome, and with gross night sleep restlessness, although the patient may not be aware of the very frequent arousals. Interview of the sleep partner, and watching the patient sleep, are both helpful for diagnosis.

A few apnoeas each night during sleep are normal physiological events in children and adults, and the frequency of these increases with age. Over 50 or more apnoeic periods of over 10 s duration during 7 h sleep are abnormal, but most patients with pathological symptomatic apnoea have hundreds of apnoeas each night. In addition to polysomnogram recording, documentation of the severity of obstructive sleep apnoea requires nocturnal blood gas studies, 24-h cardiac monitoring to detect the pattern of bradyrhythmia–tachyrhythmia that usually characterises frequent apnoeas, as well as chest X-ray and lung function studies to detect the development of the most serious complication of obstructive sleep apnoea, pulmonary hypertension and cor pulmonale secondary to repeated sleep pulmonary hypoxia. Pulmonary studies during sleep are difficult, and facilities for detailed all-night polysomnography are severely limited, so should be reserved for patient evaluation rather than initial diagnosis.

In most if not all cases of obstructive sleep apnoea, there is an anatomical abnormality of the oropharynx, and ENT assessment is essential. Lateral CT scans of the oropharynx will demonstrate a subcritical diameter during wakefulness, and this can also sometimes be shown dynamically by flow volume loop curves, which show saw-toothing on the expiratory limb. However, this abnormality is not invariably found; neither is it diagnostic.

Airway obstruction may be due to generalised fat deposition in the pickwickian syndrome, congenital and acquired anatomical deformities, focal obstruction due to lymphosarcoma or other tumour, acromegaly or myxoedema. Obstructive sleep apnoea occurs in many neuromuscular disorders, notably myotonic dystrophy, where change in chest-wall compliance aggravates the respiratory disorder. Rarely, as in multisystem atrophy, laryngeal, not oropharyngeal, obstruction is responsible for obstructive sleep apnoea. Hypnotics, alcohol, testosterone, polycythaemia, respiratory infection and anaesthetics, all make sleep apnoea worse.

Treatment of Obstructive Sleep Apnoea

Treatment is aimed at removing any predisposing cause and relieving upper airway obstruction. In some cases, weight loss, alcohol or hypnotic withdrawal, or tonsillectomy, may be curative. However, weight loss may be difficult to achieve until any respiratory obstruction is overcome.

The method of continuous positive airway pressure developed by Sullivan and his colleagues in Australia, and by many centres in North America, is now the treatment of choice for patients with symptomatic obstructive sleep apnoea who do not respond to simple remedies. Using a tight-fitting facial mask, a positive pressure of around 10 mmHg is applied to the upper airway during sleep to prevent upper airway collapse. The most crucial part of the apparatus is the mask, requiring a comfortable fit during sleep, and rubber sealants are sometimes used at the start of treatment in severe cases. Treatment with low-pressure systems can be used at home, and results in a rapid and dramatic improvement in sleep hypoxia, as well as daytime drowsiness and reversal of cor pulmonale. Also, many obese subjects previously unable to lose weight achieve this satisfactorily.

Intermittent positive airway pressure systems are also effective, although technically more complicated. Because of the success of positive pressure ventilation, the previous methods of treatment for obstructive sleep apnoea, tracheostomy and major reconstructive palatopharyngeal surgery, are no longer necessary.

Respiratory stimulant drugs (almitrine, doxapram hydrochloride) have no place in the management of obstructive sleep apnoea. These drugs first stimulate and then depress all cerebral functions, not only respiration. Daytime central nervous system stimulant drugs like amphetamine do not improve the respiratory problem at night, although the appetite-suppressant fenfluramine may help weight reduction. During sleep, the severity and frequency of apnoeic episodes is greatest during REM periods, and REM sleep suppression with protriptyline may slightly reduce the severity of sleep hypoxia in obstructive sleep apnoea. Medroxyprogesterone acetate is of limited value either as a respiratory stimulant or in causing redistribution of fat. Acetazolamide is of value in altering central chemoreceptor sensitivity to pCO_2 in patients with sleep hypoxia at high altitude, and thus in the prevention of mountain sickness.

Insomnia

Insomnia, the subjective complaint of poor, inadequate or nonrefreshing sleep, is the most common sleep disorder. The complaint of insomnia increases markedly with age. Insomnia is often the result of a short situational or emotional disturbance, medical illness or psychiatric stress, or due to a long-term combination of medical, psychological and psychiatric factors. Psychophysiological factors are of particular importance in some patients in whom a vicious circle of poor sleep, physiological activation, emotional arousal, and further fear of sleeplessness, develop.

Sleep laboratories rarely discover a hidden cause for insomnia. Surprisingly, 10%–15% of all subjects who complain of insomnia have no obvious polysomnographic abnormality. In some of these instances, the expectation of sleep may be abnormal, or minor unrecognised abnormalities of sleep structure may be present. Drug treatment (Table 7.4) for insomnia is not appropriate in most of these cases of "pseudoinsomnia".

Table 7.4. Treatment of insomnia

Insomnia	Treatment
Advanced age (N.B. benzodiazepines will increase nocturnal confusion, agitation and restlessness in some elderly patients with organic brain disease)	1. Long-acting hypnotic (nitrazepam 2.5–10 mg; flurazepam 15–30 mg). Often preferred by patients despite theoretical objections 2. "Sleep-hygiene" (jargon for regularity and comfort) 3. Audiotape (many available, particularly in North America)
Transient and situational	Analgesics Diazepam 5–15 mg
Sleep–wake cycle disturbance	Jet lag, shift work, etc.: adapt to new bedtime: take short-acting, medium-acting benzodiazepines, e.g. temazepam 10 mg, for a few nights
Short sleepers (no complaint of insomnia)	No treatment needed

"Pseudoinsomnia"
    Misinterpretation
    Delusion of sleepiness
	Observe sleep

Hypochondriasis	Explain to patient

Psychiatric disorders and insomnia
    Endogenous depression
    Anxiety–depression
        (rarely may present with hypersomnia)
	Antidepressant drug
	Sedative antidepressant
	    (use stimulant antidepressant, e.g. protriptyline)

Hypomania, mania	Neuroleptic
Parasomnia	See Table 7.3
Sleep apnoea	Relieve obstruction
Sleep myoclonus	Benzodiazepine?
Drug-induced	Withdraw CNS stimulants, coffee, tea, barbiturates, alcohol Propranolol cover if necessary
Insomnia in childhood	Consider behavioural therapy if not due to parasomnia
Insomnia in pregnancy	No drug if possible, but treat associated depressive illness if severe
Periodic insomnia	Relation to menstruation? Check endocrine disorder

Four major patterns of insomnia can be determined from the history:

1. Sleep-onset insomnia, with a sleep latency greater than 30 min. This is usually related to pain, or sudden stress such as a new baby, life events, bereavement, accident, noise, hospitalisation or stimulant drugs.

2. Sleep-maintenance insomnia. This may be combined with sleep-onset insomnia. Arousal may last for seconds or minutes, or persist for some hours. Sleep interruption may occur at specific times, as with nightmares, night terrors and cluster headaches, and frequent arousals at regular 90-min intervals are almost always due to REM sleep nightmares. This contrasts with the single night waking, usually from deep sleep and without a clear sensorium seen in NREM parasomnias (see p. 127).

3. Early morning arousal. Although this is seen with any kind of excitement, it is a specific feature of hypomania, and also endogenous depression.

4. Cyclical insomnia is mainly caused by drug abuse, alcohol dependence, or chronic medical and psychiatric disorders.

Hypnotic Drugs

Benzodiazepines

Over 8000 tons of benzodiazepines were prescribed in the United States in 1977, where as many as 4% of the population use prescription sleeping pills. All known hypnotics promote sleep and inhibit wakefulness, shorten sleep latency, and cause difficulty in arousal. All are general CNS depressants rather than specific sleep-promoting drugs. Hypnotics are only effective in the treatment of specific kinds of insomnia. Their inappropriate use in sleep apnoea will cause deterioration, not improvement. The effect of hypnotic drugs on specific sleep stages, NREM and REM sleep, are of no known clinical consequences. Benzodiazepines have replaced barbiturates on the grounds of better safety, higher effectiveness, and greater tolerance, although in overdosage benzodiazepines will cause respiratory depression. The main drawbacks to hypnotic use are rebound effects on withdrawal (these may be covered with propranolol) and daytime sedation.

Benzodiazepines all have the same actions: the difference between them arises from their differing pharmacokinetics. The most important factors (Table 7.5) which determine benzodiazepine usage in the treatment of insomnia are the individual drug dose, the bioavailability, the rate of absorption, the distribution half-life (most relevant to single-dose effects) and the elimination half-life (most relevant in chronic treatment). Sleep induction

Table 7.5. Duration of clinical effect and specific uses of selected benzodiazepine hypnotics

Drug	Dose (mg)	Duration of sedative effect (h)	Particular use
Triazolam	0.125–0.25	3–4	Onset insomnia
Temazepam	10–30	6–8	Nocturnal awakenings
Nitrazepam	2.5–10	8–12	Early morning waking
Flurazepam	15–30	Over 12	Prolonged sedation

is a function of the rate of absorption, sleep maintenance is determined by the half-life, and morning-after effects may be due to the formation of active metabolites with long half-lives. After chronic use, severe rebound insomnia is most troublesome with short-acting compounds. The rate of absorption of any benzodiazepine is slowed if given with food, and so hypnotics should be given on an empty stomach.

Amphetamine and Other Central Stimulant Drugs
(Table 7.6)

Amphetamine

Amphetamine is a basic liquid, slightly water-soluble. Amphetamine sulphate is crystalline. Absorption is rapid, with maximum plasma levels and peak clinical effects after 1–2 h. Amphetamine is a basic drug, pK_a 9.9, and 50%– 80% is excreted unchanged in the urine. Urinary excretion is pH-dependent, and an acid urine (ascorbic acid, ammonium chloride) is associated with low plasma levels and a half-life of 6–12 h, an alkaline urine (sodium bicarbonate) with high plasma levels and prolonged half-life, 24–30 h. Despite the long half-life, the alerting effect of amphetamine 5–20 mg lasts only 4–5 h.

Amphetamine causes an increase in alertness in waking subjects, and arousal from sleep, with a reduction in fatigue, increase in concentration and ability to do mental arithmetic, increase in body temperature, elevation of mood, euphoria and insomnia. Fatigue cannot be indefinitely delayed by amphetamines, and its onset may be disastrous. However, British lifeboats, by law, still carry supplies of amphetamines as a stimulant.

The behavioural responses to amphetamine depend on psychological factors. Thus, although amphetamine will improve performance in fatigued subjects or trained athletes, and cause weight loss in obesity, it has little or no effect on the ability of normally alert subjects to do mental arithmetic, the sporting achievement of untrained athletes, or appetite in narcoleptics. Although most appetite-suppressant drugs are also central nervous system stimulants, fenfluramine has little stimulant activity.

Table 7.6. Comparative effects of central stimulant drugs

Drug	Usual daily dose p.o. (mg)	Effect
Diethylpropion	75	Little cardiovascular effect
Phenmetrazine	25–75	Anorectic and stimulant
Phentermine	15–30	Mainly anorectic, mild stimulant
Fenfluramine	20–120	Little stimulant effect, and no change in REM sleep Rarely sedation, depression Onset anorectic action delayed 2 weeks
Methylphenidate	20–60	Reduction in REM sleep Stimulant and anorectic Mild peripheral action
Pemoline	20–120	Mild stimulant and anorectic effect
Prolintane	20	As pemoline
Phenylephrine	(Intranasal: oral absorption erratic)	Prominent cardiovascular actions Hypertension; reflex bradycardia Vasoconstriction Used as nasal decongestant
Hydroxyamphetamine	1% ophthalmic solution	Nonstimulant Only use as mydriatic
Methylamphetamine	5–15	Pronounced central stimulation, but may cause myocardial depression Severe drug abuse potential

Amphetamine Toxicity

Amphetamine causes tachycardia, sweating, vomiting, tremor, restlessness, chorea, headache, anxiety, systolic and diastolic hypertension, constipation, dry mouth, urinary retention, with aggressive and violent behaviour, convulsions and coma. Rarely, with large intravenous doses in addicts, subarachnoid haemorrhage and myocardial infarction have been reported. In amphetamine toxicity, ammonium chloride will increase amphetamine excretion, chlorpromazine will block peripheral and central catecholamine receptors, and nitrites or rapid-acting α-receptor antagonist drugs will lower hypertension.

Amphetamine Dependence and Abuse

Dependence and drug abuse with amphetamine and related drugs is related to the euphoriant effect. Any drug causing euphoria is open to abuse. Abuse of methylamphetamine, amphetamine and diethylpropion, has led to the restriction or control of these drugs in many countries. For example, in Australia they are considered addictive, and may only be prescribed for narcolepsy, postencephalitic parkinsonism, and in the treatment of hyperkinetic children. Abrupt withdrawal may cause severe fatigue, but physical symptoms are rare. The main danger of abuse is due to violent, aggressive behaviour. Both amphetamine and phenmetrazine are controlled in the United Kingdom by the Misuse of Drugs Act 1973.

Ephedrine

Ephedrine is an alkaloid, obtained from Chinese plants of the genus *Ephedra*, and used as a stimulant for 5000 years. The term *ma huang* or "yellow horse" refers to the colour and shape of the flowers. Ephedrine stimulates both α- and β-receptors, partly owing to release of noradrenaline, but also to a direct agonist effect. Ephedrine has a more prolonged and greater central effect than noradrenaline, causes a rise in systolic and diastolic blood pressure, sustained but mild relaxation of bronchial muscle, mydriasis without cycloplegia or increase in intraocular pressure. The central stimulant effect is less than that of amphetamine. Ephedrine has been used to treat nocturnal enuresis, both by a decrease in the depth of sleep and relaxation of the detrusor and contraction of the bladder sphincter. A few patients with myasthenia improve on ephedrine 30–90 mg daily. Ephedrine causes tolerance and dependence. Phenylpropanolamine has similar pharmacological properties to ephedrine, but has less CNS stimulant action, and is used entirely in the treatment of nasal and sinus congestion.

Mazindol

Mazindol has a different chemical structure from amphetamine. It is 5–10 times more potent as an anorectic, but 3–4 times less potent as a central stimulant. It causes little or no dependence, and has only slight abuse potential. Tolerance is uncommon. Mazindol will reduce REM sleep in doses that do not increase alertness. Like fenfluramine, mazindol increases the uptake of glucose into muscle. Side effects are similar to amphetamine, with a lower incidence. Mazindol may increase libido in women. Peak drug levels occur 2 h, and mild CNS stimulation lasts 5–6 h, following administration of mazindol 2 mg p.o. The elimination half-life is long, about 50 h.

Cocaine

Cocaine, from coca leaves, has been used for centuries in Peru and Bolivia to increase endurance and promote wellbeing, at the expense of severe dependence. This cerebrocortical stimulant effect accounts for cocaine abuse. As the dose is increased, convulsive movements and eventually tonic–clonic convulsions occur. Cocaine causes increased talkativeness, excitement, restlessness, rate of respiration, body temperature, hypertension and vomiting, and eventually death from medullary and respiratory failure. Relief of fatigue by cocaine is not due to any increase in the strength of muscle contraction, but is probably the result of reduced awareness of physical fatigue. Cocaine increases both the inhibitory and excitatory responses to noradrenaline, with blockade of noradrenaline reuptake into adrenergic nerve terminals. The most important action of cocaine is to block conduction of the nerve impulse, accounting for the local anaesthetic action.

Cocaine is a derivative of ecgonine, an amino alcohol base closely related to tropine, the amino alcohol in atropine. Synthetic local anaesthetic drugs have a similar chemical structure. The toxic effects of cocaine, and the liability to cause dependence, limit its use to surface anaesthesia of the nose and throat. In the eye it can cause sloughing of the corneal epithelium.

Caffeine and Theophylline

Sir Thomas Clifford Allbutt, the Regius Professor of Medicine at Cambridge in the early 1900s, claimed of the coffee drinker:

> The sufferer is tremulous, and loses his self-command; he is subject to fits of agitation and depression . . . he has a haggard appearance . . . As with other agents, a renewed dose of the poison gives temporary relief, but at the cost of future misery (Bowman and Rand 1980).

Caffeine and other xanthine alkaloids occur naturally in cacao, coffee beans, the West African cola nut, the guru nut chewed by the natives of the Sudan, mate and tea leaves. The cultivation of coffee began in the ninth century in the Yemen, near the town of Mocha. Cola drinks have a high caffeine content, and the daily consumption of coffee in the United States per capita is equivalent to 250 mg caffeine.

Theophylline is much more potent than caffeine as a CNS stimulant drug, and also as an inhibitor of cyclic nucleotide phosphodiesterases, whilst theobromine has little or no stimulant effect.

Increase in central monoamine turnover may account for the respiratory stimulation, increase in alertness, reduction in fatigue and more rapid and clear flow of thought due to xanthines. In addition, these drugs cause diuresis and relax smooth muscle, with a slight decrease in peripheral vascular resistance.

The absorption and distribution of theophylline p.o. when used in heart failure is unpredictable, and may lead to severe CNS toxicity, insomnia, excitement, sensory disturbance, tinnitus, sensations of flashes of light, tremor and delirium. Death following the rapid i.v. injection of aminophylline 500 mg is probably due to cardiac arrest.

Both caffeine and theophylline are rapidly and usually completely absorbed, with peak plasma levels at 1 and 2 h, respectively. Both drugs are protein-bound, with a greater concentration of caffeine than theophylline in brain and CSF than in blood. Plasma half-life of caffeine is about 3–5 h, with elimination by metabolism in the liver.

Respiratory Stimulants

Selective respiratory stimulant drugs do not exist. When most needed, in comatose patients, respiratory stimulants are ineffective in subconvulsive doses. Direct measures such as mechanical ventilation and cardiovascular support are of much more value than these drugs in the treatment of respiratory depression. However, central stimulants are of occasional value in the treatment of central alveolar hypoventilation, when hypercapnia is associated with hypoxaemia, and in acute exacerbation of ventilatory failure. These respiratory drugs should not be used in the treatment of acute sedative–hypnotic poisoning, and their frequent side effects severely limit their value in chronic obstructive airway disease.

Nonspecific respiratory stimulant drugs or analeptics stimulate the respiratory and vasomotor centres in the medulla, and increase the depth of breathing and raise the blood pressure. However, cortical as well as medullary stimulation may result in convulsions, usually followed by respiratory failure, cardiovascular collapse and death.

Doxapram

Doxapram hydrochloride (20 mg/ml: 0.5–1.5 mg/kg) will stimulate respiration and increase tidal volume by activating carotid chemoreceptors. After a single 5 mg i.v. dose, the effect lasts 5–10 min. However, side effects: hypertension, tachycardia, arrhythmias, tremor, rigidity, sweating and hyperpyrexia, are common with prolonged i.v. infusion.

Almitrine

Like doxapram, this drug is a stimulant of peripheral chemoreceptors, and may be of occasional value in the treatment of central, but not obstructive, sleep apnoea.

Acetazolamide

Acetazolamide inhibits the enzyme carbonic anhydrase, and promotes bicarbonate diuresis. This will inhibit or reverse the alkalosis of high altitude which accompanies hyperventilation and hypocapnia. It additionally causes an increase in cerebral blood flow and formation of CSF. Acetazolamide 250 mg 8-hourly generally, but not always, prevents severe acute mountain sickness. Overall, there is a reduction in periodic breathing at high altitude, a large improvement in arterial oxygenation, particularly in sleep hypoxaemia, and a reduction in pCO_2 at all levels of hypoxaemia.

The metabolic acidosis produced by acetazolamide will slow the rate of entry of potassium into muscle, and acetazolamide 250 mg 3–4 times a day will prevent attacks of muscle weakness in familial hypokalaemic periodic paralysis.

A Note on Hyperactivity in Children

Distractibility, hyperactivity, temper tantrums, irritability, aggression, disobedience, antisocial behaviour and poor concentration in children, as a result of brain damage, cerebral palsy, encephalitis, as well as emotional disturbance, may sometimes improve with the use of central stimulant drugs. Of these, methylphenidate has been most studied, on account of its mild peripheral, but marked central actions. The results are very variable. In children of normal intelligence and normal emotional adjustment, but who are hyperactive and have poor concentration, methylphenidate 5–60 mg daily (usual dose 10 mg daily) will sometimes improve concentration and diminish hyperactivity. Results are not so good with subnormal intelligence or cerebral palsy, and methylphenidate usually does not improve behaviour disorders or hyperactivity in children with severe emotional disturbance.

Notes on the Treatment of Obesity and Anorexia

Amphetamine and phenmetrazine should not be used as appetite-suppressant drugs. There is an appreciable risk of misuse or drug dependency. In any case, anorectic drugs do not cause a permanent reduction in appetite or loss of weight. Fenfluramine, phentermine, diethylpropion and mazindol are probably comparable, and will all produce a mean rate of weight loss of 200–500 g/week. Following drug withdrawal, weight regain is highly variable. They should be used with care in diabetic or hypertensive subjects. Biguanides may have a role in the treatment of obese diabetics. Overall, however, the drug treatment of obesity is poorly established. Side effects with many anorectic drugs are common, and long-term use for more than 3–6 months is not recommended.

Orexigenic (Appetite-Stimulant) Drugs

These drugs stimulate hunger, food intake, or promote weight gain, and have been used to treat anorexia. Cyproheptadine is a proven appetite stimulant; this was first shown when the drug was given to asthmatic children, who gained in weight. It increases both caloric intake and body weight. Methysergide 1 mg daily will also increase hunger, the action of these drugs indicating that serotonin may be involved in the mediation of hunger and satiety. Hunger and weight gain occur in some, but not all, psychotic patients given chlorpromazine, as well as other phenothiazines. A number of antidepressant drugs, including amitriptyline and clomipramine, cause an increase in weight in both depressed and normal subjects, suggesting this is not merely due to improvement in mood. The well-documented increase in weight during lithium prophylaxis of recurrent affective disorders probably follows lithium-induced polyuria and increased thirst rather than increased hunger.

Anorexia Nervosa

In anorexia nervosa, chlorpromazine, pimozide, insulin, antidepressants, cyproheptadine, metoclopramide, lithium and nandrolone have been used to stimulate weight gain, and clomiphene used to induce menstruation, but the effective management of anorexia depends much more on patient management, hospitalisation and nursing care, than on drug therapy.

Reference and Further Reading

Bowman WC, Rand MJ (1980) Textbook of pharmacology. Blackwell, Oxford, pp 43.1–43.51
Parkes JD (1985) Sleep and its disorders. Saunders, London

8 Immunosuppressant and Cytotoxic Drugs, Toxic and Metabolic Disorders

Non-Steroidal Immunosuppressant and Cytotoxic Drugs

Immunosuppressant drugs, including steroids, are used in many neurological disorders for which an autoimmune aetiology has been suggested. These conditions include myasthenia gravis (p. 152), polymyositis and dermatomyositis (p. 158), as well as generalised autoimmune diseases which involve the nervous system, including systemic lupus erythematosus and polyarteritis nodosa.

Many immunosuppressant drugs do not have the primary anti-inflammatory action of steroids, and do not suppress local inflammatory responses to the presence of antigen–antibody complexes. They are not of value in the treatment of cerebral oedema. Most drugs of this group owe their immunosuppressant effect to the destruction of rapidly proliferating lymphocytes involved in immune and autoimmune reactions. Because of their cytotoxic action on dividing cells they are also used in the treatment of neoplasms.

Most cytotoxic drugs are toxic to all rapidly dividing cells. Their main therapeutic as well as toxic effects in normal dosages are produced on: (a) the bone marrow and lymphoreticular tissue with reduction of formed elements of blood, and with immunosuppression giving rise to superinfection; (b) the gastrointestinal mucosa, with stomatitis, diarrhoea, haemorrhage and septicaemia; (c) the hair follicles, with alopecia; (d) the testes, with sterility and mutations; (e) the foetus, with teratogenesis and abortion. These drugs are also oncogenic and may induce tumours at sites other than those being treated. All these drugs delay wound healing.

Rapid breakdown of neoplastic tissue produced by some of these drugs may cause hyperuricaemia and consequent renal damage. This can be prevented by giving allopurinol. However, mercaptopurine and thioguanine are metabolised by xanthine oxidase, and blockade of this enzyme by allopurinol increases the toxicity of mercaptopurine, thioguanine and their thioether derivatives azathioprine and thiamiprine.

Cyclophosphamide

Cyclophosphamide is a nitrogen mustard derivative which replaces hydrogen atoms on accessible DNA molecules with an alkyl group, damaging the molecule. The effect on DNA is similar to that of X-rays. Cyclophosphamide is mainly used in the treatment of neoplastic disease, including Hodgkin's disease, leukaemia and myeloma.

Cyclophosphamide is well absorbed orally, with peak plasma level at 1 h. It is distributed throughout the extracellular fluid, and subsequently into cells. Less than 10% is protein-bound in plasma. Cyclophosphamide is largely metabolised by the hepatic microsomal mixed-oxidase system to nontoxic metabolites, with a half-life of 4–6 h. Between 10% and 30% is excreted unchanged in urine. Cyclophosphamide may interact additively with other cytotoxic drugs with a different mode of action.

Methotrexate

Methotrexate is a folic acid analogue used in the treatment of meningeal leukaemia. Methotrexate exerts its antifolic action by binding with high affinity to dihydrofolate reductase, causing a deficiency of the tetrahydrofolate needed for the synthesis of thymidylic acid from deoxuridylic acid. This action is cytotoxic to rapidly dividing cells, particularly in the gastrointestinal tract, bone marrow and foetus.

Methotrexate is well absorbed intramuscularly. In small doses it is well absorbed orally, but higher doses are less well absorbed, perhaps because of their gastrointestinal toxicity. In plasma, 25%–50% is protein-bound, and methotrexate competes with sulphonamides and salicylates for binding sites. Penetration into CSF is poor, so for carcinomatous meningitis or meningeal leukaemia it is given intrathecally. It is excreted largely (80%) unchanged in urine, with a half-life of 28 h. Methotrexate effects are antagonised by folinic acid.

Azathioprine

Azathioprine is a purine analogue which slowly releases 6-mercaptopurine in the body. It is of value in the treatment of myasthenia gravis and polymyositis. 6-Mercaptopurine replaces normal purines in the cell, forming an active ribose-5-phosphate derivative which inhibits cellular reactions, perhaps because of its resemblance to ATP. Azathioprine is cytotoxic to rapidly dividing cells, and reduces lymphocytic antibody production.

Peak plasma azathioprine levels occur 2 h after oral dosage, and 6-mercaptopurine is then released slowly. Azathioprine is about 30% bound to plasma protein. The 6-mercaptopurine released enters cells rapidly. So while the plasma half-life of azathioprine is 3–5 h, that of 6-mercaptopurine is only 20–50 min. Most of a dose of azathioprine is biotransformed into nucleotides, or by oxidation to thiouric acid. Only about 1% of a dose of azathioprine appears in the urine as 6-mercaptopurine. Oxidation to thiouric acid is inhibited by allopurinol, which increases the cytotoxic effect of azathioprine.

Vinca Alkaloids (Vincristine, Vinblastine)

Obtained from the periwinkle plant, these drugs act like colchicine by inhibition of mitosis in metaphase, through disruption of the microtubular spindle. They also impair uridine incorporation into RNA. They are used, sometimes in combination with nitrosoureas, steroids and radiotherapy, in the treatment of malignant gliomas. They are given i.v. not more than once a week, because of their toxic effects rather than any pharmacokinetic consideration. They do not cross the intact blood–brain barrier. The serum half-life of vincristine is about 2 h, that of vinblastine 3 h. Dose-related toxic effects are as for other cytotoxic drugs, with the addition of a severe sensorimotor neuropathy attributable to their effect in disrupting microtubular systems in neurones. Vinblastine has been reported to be relatively free from embryonic and teratogenic effects, although it is hard to see how this could be true.

Wilson's Disease

The liver and brain injury occurring in Wilson's disease is due to copper excess and, if this excess can be removed soon enough, the patient can usually return to normal life. However, it has been estimated that the correct diagnosis is made in only one-quarter of all those with the disease, which in any case is uncommon, with approximately 2000 diagnosed cases in the United Kingdom.

Wilson's disease presents with a purely psychiatric illness in 20% of cases, with unexplained liver disease, hepatosplenomegaly, hypersplenism or attacks of jaundice in 50%, and with signs of brain failure, tremor, clumsiness, ataxia, rigidity, failure of school work, epilepsy, sleep disorder or dementia, in the remainder. In a very small minority, the first signs are those of renal or bone disease. If the correct diagnosis is not made, and treatment is not given, all these patients are doomed to die in coma, in terminal liver disease, mute, immobile or demented.

The biochemical diagnosis of Wilson's disease depends on the following findings:

1. The plasma coeruloplasmin level is usually, but not always low (below 20 μg per 100 ml) with low serum copper levels (less than 80 μg/ml).

2. Urinary copper excretion is high (over 100 μg radioactive copper per 24 h). However, high urinary copper output also occurs in biliary cirrhosis.

3. The liver copper content is very high (above 250 μg/g on needle biopsy) with, on histology, a positive stain for copper.

4. There is an overall diminution of copper incorporation into coeruloplasmin, with a prolonged turnover of body copper.

5. All cases with neurological involvement are said to have a rusty brown Kayser–Fleischer ring in the corneoscleral junction.

Treatment of Wilson's Disease

Effective body de-coppering can be established in a number of ways. Both penicillamine, a metabolite of penicillin, and the possibly less toxic alternative trientine, act as chelating agents. Zinc will increase gastrointestinal copper loss. Molybdate has recently been used with success. Also, dietary copper reduction may be helpful, although avoiding high copper content foods such as shellfish, liver and chocolate is not essential.

The ultimate response to treatment is often excellent, although clinical improvement is sometimes slow. In most instances, renal tubular defects, liver disease, and neurological problems, all slowly improve, as do CT scan appearances. However, in some cases, despite improvement in liver disease, the initial neurological response is poor, or neurological deterioration may apparently accelerate on commencing penicillamine. The best course here is to persevere with treatment, and possibly combine penicillamine with zinc and dietary copper restriction.

Penicillamine

Penicillamine is the amino acid β,β-dimethylcysteine found in penicillin hydrolysates. As well as in Wilson's disease, penicillamine is used in severe active or progressive rheumatoid arthritis, chronic active hepatitis, primary biliary cirrhosis, scleroderma and in cystinuria.

Actions of penicillamine include:

1. Chelation of copper, mercury, zinc and lead, and promotion of urinary excretion of these metals. The stability of chelate complexes of penicillamine with copper exceeds that of endogenous coeruloplasmin.

2. Inhibition of release of lysosomal enzymes in connective tissue.

3. Dissociation of macroglobulins in autoimmune disease.

4. Inhibition of various enzymes for which pyridoxine is a cofactor. A case of optic neuritis, due to penicillamine and responsive to pyridoxine, has been reported.

5. Formation from cystine of the more water-soluble penicillamine cysteine disulphide.

(+)-Penicillamine is well absorbed orally, unlike other chelating agents. The half-life is about 7 h, and urinary excretion is rapid. Penicillamine 1 g daily results in the excretion of about 2 mg copper as the penicillamine–copper chelate, although the in vitro capacity of this amount is 200 mg copper.

Penicillamine Toxicity

(+)-Penicillamine must be continued for life, and acute sensitivity, as well as delayed toxic reactions, are common. (+)-Penicillamine itself is relatively nontoxic, and much of the toxicity reported is due to the use of (−)- or (±)-forms.

A quarter of patients develop skin rashes, arthritis, fever and lymphadenopathy in the first 1–2 weeks of penicillamine treatment. These usually improve on drug withdrawal, after which low-dosage penicillamine can be restarted, and the dose gradually increased. Disturbance of taste is very common during early treatment, but usually resolves. Allergic rashes in the first 12 weeks of treatment may respond to cyproheptadine and penicillamine dose reduction. Arthralgia or fever may respond to temporary dosage reduction or prednisolone 30 mg daily. The nephrotic syndrome, neutropenia, thrombocytopenia, a lupus-like syndrome, and optic neuropathy, as well as Goodpasture's syndrome, are more serious toxic effects of penicillamine that may develop for the first time after chronic therapy.

In probably fewer than 5% of patients treatment with penicillamine becomes unacceptable. The development of a lupus-like syndrome, or the nephrotic syndrome, requires the drug to be stopped. After about 6 months, some 20% of patients develop persistent proteinuria, accompanied by microscopic haematuria. If heavy or increasing proteinuria occurs, penicillamine should be totally withdrawn.

Iron deficiency anaemia and haemolytic anaemia may be produced with prolonged treatment. Thrombocytopenia and neutropenia may occur at any time. Penicillamine should be withdrawn with platelet count below 120 000 per mm^3, or neutropenia below 2000 per mm^3. Recovery is usually rapid, and low-dosage (250 mg daily) penicillamine may be restarted.

Stomatitis, various skin lesions including pemphigus, and a myasthenic syndrome, can occur with long-term use. (+)-Penicillamine may cause muscle fatigue, with electrophysiological findings typical of myasthenia, and improvement in weakness with rest and anticholinesterases.

During penicillamine treatment, white blood cell and platelet counts, and urine tests for protein and blood, should be done weekly in the first 6 weeks and then monthly. Acetylpenicillamine, the N-acetyl derivative of (+)-penicillamine, may produce fewer side effects.

Trientine

Trientine (triethylenetetramine dihydrochloride) 400–800 mg three times daily, has been developed by Walsh as an alternative treatment for patients with Wilson's disease who show immunological intolerance or toxicity with penicillamine. Trientine is an effective oral chelating agent, and may be less toxic than penicillamine. As with penicillamine, blood and urinary copper levels fall sharply, and neurological improvement is often striking. Immune complex nephritis and platelet and white cell dyscrasias on penicillamine may not recur with trientine. Both drugs occasionally produce a systemic lupus erythematosus syndrome (Walsh 1982).

Zinc

Large oral doses of zinc result in a negative copper balance in patients with Wilson's disease (Brewer et al. 1983). The clinical effectiveness of zinc has not yet been fully established. It is not clear how zinc promotes increased faecal copper excretion. Brewer suggested that this may be due to an increase in synthesis of the metal-binding protein metallothionein in the intestine, resulting in the binding of both endogenous and dietary copper, and subsequent elimination with mucosal sloughing. Since much of the toxicity of penicillamine is dose-related, the combination of zinc with low-dose penicillamine therapy may be valuable. In contrast to the effect of penicillamine, the increased copper excretion resulting from zinc therapy is primarily faecal, and does not commence for several days after starting treatment.

Heavy Metal Poisoning

Two derivatives of ethylenediamine are used clinically as chelating agents in the treatment of heavy metal toxicity: calcium disodium edetate (EDTA) and calcium trisodium pentetate. The main clinical use of EDTA is in the treatment of acute lead poisoning and lead encephalopathy. Slow i.v. infusion of 1 g in 0.5 l over 1 h will remove 3–5 mg lead.

The search for an antidote against arsenic, which reacts with SH groups, led to the production of British anti-lewisite (dimercaprol, BAL) and a sulphonated derivative, unithiol, in the Soviet Union. These compounds compete with tissue SH groups for arsenic. Dimercaprol is used in the treatment of arsenic, antimony, mercury and gold poisoning. However, it does not reduce concentrations of mercury in the brain, and is ineffective in the treatment of human brain damage from methyl mercury. Also, dimercaprol–iron chelates are more toxic than iron, and EDTA, not BAL, should be used in acute iron poisoning.

Dimercaprol is given i.m. in a 5%–10% solution in arachis oil. Peak concentrations occur at 30–60 min, and the drug is rapidly metabolised and excreted. Early treatment is essential. Dimercaprol produces alarming rather than serious side effects, with severe feelings of anxiety and unrest and dose-related hypertension, tachycardia, nausea, headache, sweating and abdominal pain.

Alcoholism

Perhaps 5% of the adult population of the United Kingdom drink enough alcohol to interfere with their health. The management of liver and brain disease, due to alcohol, particularly in young males, is of increasing importance.

Ethyl alcohol is completely and rapidly absorbed from the gastrointestinal tract. Hepatic metabolism is limited to approximately 7–10 g/h, and is more rapid in habitual than in occasional drinkers. The major immediate effect of alcohol on the central nervous system is depression of mental and motor function. In nonhabituated subjects, a blood level of 30 mg per 100 ml is associated with mild euphoria; 50 mg per 100 ml produces mild incoordination; 100 mg per 100 ml, ataxia; 300 mg per 100 ml, stupor; and 400–500 mg per 100 ml, death.

Chronic Effects of Alcohol on the Brain

Alcoholism may cause hepatic encephalopathy, Wernicke's encephalopathy, and a specific alcoholic dementia, as well as result in head injury.

Severe chronic hepatic encephalopathy results in a wide range of features, with poor concentration, poor memory, slurred speech, drowsiness, ataxia, asterixis with hepatic foetor, and prominent frontal EEG slow activity ("slow rollers"). All these may be present despite well-compensated liver disease. The precise way in which liver coma is induced is still uncertain, although the presence of a naturally created or surgical portal-systemic shunt, changes in nitrogen metabolism, amino acid imbalance, and false neurotransmitters produced by failure of hepatic detoxification, have all been implicated.

The connection between hepatic encephalopathy and nitrogen metabolism is undisputed, and ammonium salts will cause encephalopathy and raise blood ammonia levels in patients with cirrhosis. However, plasma ammonia levels correlate poorly with the degree of encephalopathy. Nitrogenous toxins are partly derived from bacterial action in the intestine, and bowel cleaning, with a low-protein diet, neomycin or other broad-spectrum antibiotic and lactulose, is well established. Lactulose, or the less sugary lactulose derivative lactilol, combined with restriction of dietary protein, remains the mainstay of treatment for chronic hepatic encephalopathy. Lactulose acidifies the gastrointestinal contents, reduces ammonia absorption, and is a laxative.

Other theories to account for the occurrence of encephalopathy and liver disease have stressed the role of amino acid imbalance, with an increase in aromatic and decrease in branched-chain amino acids in the blood in hepatic encephalopathy. There is no conclusive evidence for the theory that encephalopathy is due to reduction in cerebral dopamine or noradrenaline levels associated with catecholamine receptor blockade by false neurotransmitters, although bromocriptine 15 mg daily has been reported to cause an overall improvement in memory and motor function, as well as an increase in the EEG dominant frequency, increase in cerebral blood flow, oxygen consumption, and glucose utilisation in chronic hepatic encephalopathy, despite no change in blood ammonia levels. This action of bromocriptine has not been confirmed, and the drug must be introduced slowly, and often causes vomiting.

Wernicke's encephalopathy is characterised by thiamine deficiency, with disordered consciousness, ophthalmoplegia and ataxia. Minor degrees of thiamine deficiency may be converted to full-blown Wernicke's encephalopathy by the administration of glucose without added thiamine (see p. 216). A peripheral neuropathy is often present, and Korsakoff's psychosis may develop, although the reason for this, whether metabolic, neurophysiological or genetic, is still unclear. However, thiamine triphosphate appears to be necessary for the stability of nerve membranes and impulse conduction, as well as for transketolase reactions.

Chronic alcoholism causes brain damage, independent of liver disease or thiamine deficiency, and brain damage is sometimes an early presentation of alcoholism. Pathological examination of the brains of young alcoholics sometimes reveals unsuspected cerebral atrophy, often most marked in the frontal areas. There is some correlation between cortical and cerebellar atrophy. In chronic alcoholics, intellectual decline may be more severe than liver damage, and mental deterioration can occur without biochemical evidence of severe hepatic disease. The results of psychometric testing do not necessarily correlate with liver function studies or the CT scan appearance. However, CT scans in alcoholics have revealed a surprisingly high proportion of cerebral atrophy as well as central and cerebellar atrophy.

The cause of cortical atrophy in alcoholics is quite unknown. If alcohol does have a direct cytotoxic effect on cortical neurones, then the therapeutic possibilities are limited to prevention, not treatment. Symptoms such as fatigue, loss of the ability for abstract thought, emotional immaturity, sleep disturbances and sleep apnoea, may all contribute to the overall intellectual decline. Complete abstinence for a prolonged period may cause a partial reversal of symptoms.

Delirium Tremens

Delirium tremens is the most dramatic and grave of all alcohol complications, with a mortality of 10%–15%, although it is usually a short-term problem, with recovery in 72 h. The condition usually follows a drinking bout in alcoholics. Most patients have a high pulse rate, high blood pressure and fever, with intense perspiration, dilated pupils, severe tremor of the limbs, nausea, vomiting and other gastrointestinal disturbances, as well as intense hallucinosis.

The symptoms of alcohol intoxication and delirium tremens are different, and plasma alcohol levels are not always high in delirium tremens. Also, alcohol will usually abolish, at least temporarily, tremulousness and hallucinations. In some, but not all, patients with delirium tremens, plasma magnesium concentrations are low, and should be restored to normal, although the occurrence of hypomagnesaemia does not explain the onset of delirium tremens.

Withdrawal symptoms in delirium tremens can be minimised by benzodiazepines or chlormethiazole, which act quickly and reduce agitation without serious depression of respiration. Any intercurrent illness or infection associated with or precipitating alcohol withdrawal should be treated. Dehydration, potassium depletion and alcoholic ketoacidosis are often severe, and may require up to 6000 ml fluid replacement daily, of which 1500 ml should be normal saline.

Severe liver damage results in hypoglycaemia, and starvation may result in ketoacidosis. Thiamine (50 mg i.v.) should be given before glucose. Sympathetic overactivity, palpitations and hypertension in delirium tremens may be controlled with propranolol. Rum fits probably do not need prophylaxis or treatment, although the possibility that withdrawal fits are associated with head injury, subdural haematoma, metabolic disorders or meningitis, and aggravated by electrolyte and acid–base disturbance, must be considered. Not infrequently, alcohol withdrawal results in status epilepticus.

Rum fits in alcoholics usually occur in the immediate 6- to 48-h period after alcohol withdrawal, and are to be distinguished from the seizures of idiopathic epilepsy that are undoubtedly more common after fairly minor alcohol consumption (not severe alcoholism). Rum fits have several distinctive features, with a burst of one or two generalised, not focal, seizures in the period of early alcohol withdrawal, but a normal interictal EEG recording, and no greater liability to seizures at other times than in the nondrinking population. Withdrawal seizures can be prevented by prophylactic phenytoin, although benzodiazepines alone are usually adequate. Generalised or partial seizures in alcoholics are often related to head injury, anoxia or ischaemia, as well as to alcohol withdrawal.

Treatment of Alcoholism

Total abstinence is probably necessary for the successful treatment of alcoholism. The patient needs to recognise that he or she is an alcoholic, and must desire to be helped. This may require pressure from the family and the employer as well as the physician. A rough index of the patient's willingness to give up alcohol is given by the degree of compliance with daily disulfiram prophylaxis. The single most effective force in dealing with the problem of alcoholism is probably Alcoholics Anonymous.

References

Brewer GJ, Hill GM, Prasad AS, Cossack ZT, Rabbani P (1983) Oral zinc therapy for Wilson's disease. Arch Intern Med 99: 314–320

Walsh JM (1982) Treatment of Wilson's disease with trientine (triethylene tetramine). Lancet I: 643–647

9 Treatment of Diseases of Nerve and Muscle

Introduction

Primary muscle disease causes muscle wasting and weakness without sensory change. Disease of the muscle end-plate, myasthenia, causes fatiguable muscle weakness without wasting (at least until the late stages of the illness). Peripheral nerve diseases cause muscle wasting and weakness with peripheral sensory deficit. Unfortunately, many diseases affecting muscles and nerves are not susceptible to specific treatment. However, the resulting weakness and wasting, and sensory change if present, require appropriate symptomatic therapy and the use of mechanical aids. This general management of muscle wasting and weakness will be discussed first.

Amongst the diseases under consideration, myasthenia gravis, inflammatory muscle disease, and the acute and chronic forms of demyelinating peripheral neuropathy can be treated successfully. These illnesses will be discussed separately.

General Management

Muscle wasting, whether due to primary muscle disease or peripheral neuropathy, is often associated with contractures. A typical example is the contracture of calf muscles that causes tightness of the Achilles tendon and fixed plantar flexion of the foot. Physiotherapy in the form of passive exercises is essential to prevent contractures.

Much effort has been expended in attempting to show that electrical stimulation of wasted or denervated muscle can promote increased power. However, such a form of treatment has not been shown to be effective.

The functional disability produced by muscle weakness can be assisted by mechanical aids. For example, a below-knee splint activated by a toe spring can be used to dorsiflex the ankle during walking, or a cock-up wrist splint can extend the wrist and fingers to allow useful grip. Simple orthotic devices can be used to improve function as, for example, a lightweight plastic ankle splint holding the ankle at 90°.

Sensory loss due to peripheral neuropathy may cause skin ulceration, particularly in diabetics. Scrupulous attention to skin care and daily examination of pressure points is essential in this situation. Specially moulded boots may be required to relieve pressure and prevent ulcers. Some forms of peripheral neuropathy affect not only the somatic nerves, but also the autonomic nervous system. In such patients, postural hypotension and sphincter disturbances may require symptomatic treatment (see Chap. 10).

Myasthenia Gravis

Myasthenia gravis has now been established as due to an autoimmune response to the acetylcholine receptor on the muscle end-plate. The reason for such an autoimmune attack is not known, but may involve an abnormal response of the thymus to the acetylcholine receptor antigen, resulting in the generation of a forbidden clone of T cells which provokes the formation of anti-acetylcholine receptor antibodies. Correlation between the titre of anti-acetylcholine receptor antibodies and disease severity in myasthenia gravis is poor. Normal antibody titres do not rule out myasthenia gravis, particularly in those with localised ocular myasthenia, but also in some acute cases of generalised disease; nor do normal antibody findings exclude the possibility of a successful response to treatment. Anti-acetylcholine titres may be similar in both good and poor responders to, for example, steroid therapy. However, it is not infrequent to find very high titres associated with severe, generalised myasthenia and a good response to treatment. A proportion of those with myasthenia gravis have a thymic tumour (thymoma) or thymic hyperplasia, and thymectomy is an established aid in the management of myasthenia gravis. Plasmapheresis may be used to remove anti-acetylcholine receptor antibodies. Finally, the muscle weakness of myasthenia gravis may be alleviated by anticholinesterase drugs, which prevent the breakdown of acetylcholine at the muscle end-plate receptor, thereby enhancing neuromuscular transmission.

Symptomatic Treatment

The majority of patients with myasthenia gravis require anticholinesterase drugs, despite other forms of treatment. The two most useful agents are neostigmine and pyridostigmine. The oral dose of neostigmine and of pyridostigmine is 30 times higher than the intramuscular dose. There is a large variation in individual patient sensitivity to these cholinergic drugs. Their dosage must be adjusted according to the patient's response. Doses in children are particularly variable, so that very small doses should be given to commence with, then slowly increased depending upon the response. Tailoring of individual dosage is crucial in each patient. There is a critical point of maximum therapeutic effectiveness with optimal muscle strength, but without side effects, particularly the common gastrointestinal disturbances or, more seriously, the fasciculation and paralysis of voluntary muscle. Anticholinesterase drugs are not usually required at night.

Neostigmine causes improvement for up to 4 h. Pyridostigmine requires a higher dosage, but has a slightly more prolonged action. Management is simpler if only one drug is given; any overlap in action of several drugs only complicates dosage schedules.

For the patient with moderately severe myasthenia, average doses would be:

1. Neostigmine: 15–45 mg p.o. at 3- to 4-hourly intervals
2. Pyridostigmine: 60–180 mg p.o. at 4-hourly intervals
3. Ambenonium: 5–40 mg p.o. daily at 4- to 6-hourly intervals

The longer-acting compounds may be useful in patients whose muscles are weak on waking.

Routine administration of anticholinergic drugs to prevent colic or excessive salivation is unnecessary. Anticholinergics may mask the parasympathetic symptoms of excessive gastrointestinal stimulation, and delay recognition of potentially serious overdosage. Side effects can sometimes be avoided by giving smaller doses of anticholinesterases frequently. In any case, tolerance to parasympathetic stimulation sometimes develops with prolonged treatment.

Anticholinesterase Drugs

Acetylcholine was historically the first neurotransmitter substance to be recognised. Acetylcholine is an unstable ester of choline and acetic acid. It is synthesised in cholinergic nerve terminals by the enzyme choline acetyl transferase, which transfers the acetyl group to choline from acetyl coenzyme A. Choline comes from the diet, and lecithin in the diet is a source of choline. The release of acetylcholine from storage vesicles is calcium-dependent and blocked by botulinus toxin.

Acetylcholine receptors are of two main types, nicotinic (N) and muscarinic (M). N receptors are in the neuromuscular junction of skeletal muscle. M receptors are in the parasympathetic nervous system. Nicotine is obtained from tobacco. Muscarine is the active principle of the poisonous mushroom *Amanita muscaria*, which is chewed, dried, in Eastern Siberia. It causes a stimulant effect which is due to muscimol (a GABA agonist) rather than to muscarine. The stimulant effect is repeated by drinking urine.

In different cholinergic synapses, there are marked differences in ultra-structure, distribution of acetylcholinesterases and speed of neurotransmission. The discrete neuromuscular ending has little similarity with the hundred thousand or so ganglion cells which are closely packed in the superior cervical ganglion.

Acetylcholine released from nerve endings stimulates both N and M receptors. This causes: in the heart slowing of contraction; in blood vessels vasodilatation; in exocrine glands secretion of saliva, bronchial mucus and sweat; in the intestines constriction and peristalsis with intestinal cramp and pain; in the urinary system ureteric and bladder constriction; in the eye ciliary muscle contraction causing relaxation of the lens which is then focused for near vision, contraction of the iris circular muscle resulting in pupillary constriction and a reduction of elevated intraocular pressure.

N receptor stimulation causes physiological contraction of skeletal muscle as well as initial stimulation and subsequent blockade of cholinergic receptors and autonomic ganglia. With different drugs, the N:M stimulation ratio may vary. Thus pyridostigmine has less gastrointestinal effect than neostigmine for an equal effect in myasthenia.

The central effects of anticholinesterase drugs are determined by their chemical nature. Physostigmine, but not neostigmine or pyridostigmine, will penetrate the brain. Plasma (pseudo) cholinesterase is not associated with cholinergic terminals, but occurs in many areas of the nervous system and liver, as well as in the plasma. Inhibitors of acetylcholinesterase act at all sites accessible to the drug, and may cause reversible (e.g. physostigmine) or irreversible (e.g. the organophosphorus derivative diisopropylfluoro-phosphate, DFP) inactivation of the enzyme.

Physostigmine (eserine, an alkaloid which occurs in the Calabar bean) is highly lipid-soluble, and given orally easily enters the CNS. Physostigmine does not act on tissues whose postganglionic parasympathetic nerves have been made to degenerate. Large doses produce headache, bradycardia, cardiac arrest and respiratory failure.

Neostigmine and pyridostigmine are synthetic anticholinesterases. Pyridostigmine 60 mg is equivalent to neostigmine 15 mg. Both drugs are poorly lipid-soluble, poorly absorbed by mouth, so that the parenteral dose is less than 1/30 of the oral dose. Neostigmine is rapidly inactivated in the gut, but has a more rapid absorption and onset of effect than pyridostigmine. Absorption is better from the intestine than from the stomach, where the acid environment tends to keep the drug molecules ionised. Both are subject to first-pass hepatic metabolism; hydrolysis products of anticholinesterases appear in the urine.

Orally administered pyridostigmine appears in the blood 0.5–1 h after dosing, with peak plasma levels at 1.5–2 h. With neostigmine, the clinical effect occurs within 30 min of oral dosing. For optimal clinical response, peak plasma pyridostigmine levels are between 45 and 85 mg/ml. To achieve these levels, there may be an 11-fold difference in oral dosage.

Edrophonium is another synthetic anticholinesterase which has a very short duration of action (5–10 min) for it is rapidly taken up in the circulation by the liver and kidneys. It is employed as a diagnostic test for myasthenia gravis. An initial bolus of 2 mg is given intravenously, followed by a further 8 mg about 1 min later. Patients with myasthenia gravis will show dramatic improvement in muscle fatiguability and strength.

Ambenonium and distigmine are longer-acting synthetic anticholinesterases. Distigmine (Ubretid) is a longer-acting variant of pyridostigmine which does not cross the blood–brain barrier, and which has found a place in the treatment of bladder disorders.

Anticholinesterase Toxicity: Cholinergic Crisis

Overdosage of drugs used to treat myasthenia gravis may cause anticholinesterase toxicity and a cholinergic crisis. This results in miosis, lachrymation, sweating and salivation, bradycardia, hypotension, gastrointestinal pain, and very occasionally cardiac arrest and bronchospasm. In normal subjects there is prominent muscle fasciculation. In patients with myasthenia gravis, there is a dangerous cholinergic paralysis of skeletal muscle.

The signs and symptoms of anticholinesterase overdosage in myasthenia gravis vary considerably. A cholinergic crisis can usually be differentiated from the weakness and paralysis of a worsening myasthenic state by the additional signs of parasympathetic stimulation; epigastric discomfort, abdominal pain, diarrhoea and vomiting, excessive salivation, pallor, cold sweating, urinary urgency and blurred vision. The pupils are dilated, there may be an increase in blood pressure with or without bradycardia, and there is usually severe anxiety and panic. The usual features distinguishing cholinergic crisis from myasthenic crisis, both of which cause paralysis, are that the overdosed patient is "wet", with profuse sweating, salivation, and bubbly lungs, and the pupils are dilated.

Edrophonium is said to be of value in determining whether a patient with myasthenia is receiving too little or too much anticholinesterase therapy. If treatment is excessive, an injection of edrophonium has no effect or may increase weakness. If the patient is underdosed, edrophonium improves muscle strength. However, different muscles are often affected in opposite ways in an individual patient. Thus, limb muscles may be underdosed and improve with the edrophonium, while respiratory muscles may be overdosed and get worse. Thus, edrophonium may give a false answer, depending on which part of the body is examined, and may even be dangerous if there is selective cholinergic overdosage of respiratory or laryngeal muscles.

In someone suspected of a cholinergic crisis, the safest management is immediately to preserve respiration, by tracheal intubation and artificial respiration. All anticholinesterase drugs should be withdrawn and the patient tested with edrophonium at daily intervals to establish when anticholinesterase sensitivity returns, at which time anticholinesterase treatment can be reintroduced. A cholinergic crisis is indeed a medical emergency and it is far better to take action early rather than late. Signs of incipient respiratory failure are increasing respiration and pulse rates in an anxious, distressed patient. These changes occur well in advance of alterations in blood gas concentrations, which indicate that respiratory failure has been allowed to occur.

Another major problem in the management of myasthenics is their treatment during surgery or labour. In these circumstances replacement of oral anticholinesterase treatment by 1/30 of the same dose given intravenously or intramuscularly at 2- to 4-hourly intervals, as determined by the clinical state and vital capacity, is required until drugs can be given again by mouth.

Drug Interactions

Patients with myasthenia gravis are very sensitive to many drugs and the effects of anticholinesterase may be reduced or prevented by:

1. Tubocurarine and other neuromuscular blocking drugs. The myasthenic's sensitivity may be increased 100-fold by curare, gallamine or pancuronium.

2. Depolarising neuromuscular blocking drugs.

3. Aminoglycoside antibiotics (e.g. gentamicin), which have some curariform action and impair conduction in terminal nerve fibres.

4. Other antibiotics such as polymyxin, colistin and bacitracin.

5. Respiratory depressants, such as barbiturates and benzodiazepines.

6. Local anaesthetics, including beta-blockers and antiarrhythmia drugs, which reduce the excitability of muscle membranes. These include lignocaine, procainamide and propranolol.

7. Hypokalaemic agents, digitalis and diuretics. Quinine, quinidine (tonic water) may cause decompensation.

Treatment of the Cause of Myasthenia Gravis

Thymectomy has been shown to be an effective method of inducing a remission of myasthenia gravis in 80% of younger patients. Thus, thymectomy is now considered the treatment of choice in patients with generalised myasthenia who are otherwise healthy under the age of about 50 years. Both males and females will respond. Thymectomy is not required for localised ocular myasthenia. In subjects with thymic tumours, management is difficult and preliminary DXT may be indicated. Most of these tumours are locally malignant, but do not metastasise.

Steroids are indicated for both young and old patients with myasthenia gravis. A period of steroid treatment may be used in the young to prepare the patient for subsequent thymectomy. Steroids are the treatment of choice in those over the age of about 50 years.

High-dose prednisolone (60–100 mg daily) will produce improvement of myasthenia gravis within 2 weeks of starting therapy, but increased weakness, occasionally provoking a myasthenic crisis, can occur within 2–10 days of starting each treatment. It is therefore wiser to begin with a low-dose, alternate-day steroid regime (prednisolone 25 mg alternate days, gradually increasing the dosage by 10 mg at weekly intervals until an alternate-day dosage of 60–100 mg is achieved). This method avoids initial weakness, but full benefit takes 2–4 months to establish. The maintenance dose of prednisolone can often then be reduced to some 15–30 mg on alternate days. Most patients require long-term steroid therapy, so need careful observation for infection, hypokalaemia, or other complications of long-term steroid treatment. For this reason, azathioprine (1–5 mg/kg daily in adults; usual dosage 100–150 mg per 24 h) may be employed in conjunction with alternate-day steroid treatment to reduce the complications of long-term steroid therapy. The response to azathioprine in myasthenia gravis is slower than that to steroid therapy alone, and may take at least 3–6 months to appear.

Azathioprine is a cytotoxic immunosuppressant widely used to prevent rejection in organ transplant recipients. It is also used to treat a wide variety of autoimmune and collagen disorders. Azathioprine is metabolised to mercaptopurine which inhibits DNA synthesis and replication. The drug is inactivated by xanthine oxidase and is excreted in the urine. Xanthine oxidase inhibition (e.g. allopurinol), and renal disease markedly increase toxicity of azathioprine. In addition to marrow suppression, the most important toxicity of azathioprine is hepatic, so patients require regular blood counts and tests of liver function throughout treatment. Azathioprine produces a high incidence of abortion, although major congenital malformations are uncommon in those babies that do come to term. Accordingly, azathioprine should not be used in the control of myasthenia in patients of childbearing age.

Plasmapheresis, by removing anti-acetylcholine receptor antibodies, may produce a temporary remission in myasthenia gravis. Plasma exchange of 5%–6% of body weight per week for up to ten exchanges is effective. The use of plasmapheresis in myasthenia gravis is limited to patients with severe illness, or during pregnancy, or whilst waiting for other forms of therapy to become effective.

The Myasthenic Syndrome

The myasthenic syndrome (or the Lambert–Eaton syndrome) also presents with fatiguable muscle weakness, but has a different physiological, pharmacological and pathological basis from myasthenia gravis. Frequently, but not always, it is associated with the presence of carcinoma, particularly of the lung. Patients complain of fatigue and muscle weakness, but eye movements are usually spared. Characteristically, the tendon jerks are unobtainable, but appear when the tendons are tapped repeatedly. This is analogous to the diagnostic electrophysiological findings of increased muscle potential potentiation on repetitive stimulation (the reverse occurs in myasthenia gravis, the muscle action potential getting smaller on repetitive nerve stimulation). There is some recent evidence to suggest that the myasthenic syndrome, like myasthenia gravis, may be immunologically determined; a few patients have responded to plasmapheresis or immunosuppressant therapy.

The myasthenic syndrome is not helped by anticholinesterase drugs, but can respond to guanidine hydrochloride (0.75–2 g p.o. daily). Guanidine is a strong base, freely water-soluble, with presynaptic rather than postsynaptic actions. It causes an increase in acetylcholine release and response to nerve stimuli. (Caffeine has similar, but less marked, effects at presynaptic motor nerve terminals.) In high dosage guanidine is toxic, causing hypotension and atrial fibrillation, bone marrow depression, renal tubular necrosis, interstitial neuritis, irritability, ataxia and confusion. Other drugs reported to cause improvement in the myasthenic syndrome include calcium salts, tetraethylammonium, and 4-aminopyridine, all of which enhance neurotransmitter output.

Inflammatory Muscle Disease

Polymyositis, with or without skin changes (dermatomyositis) occurs in the setting of a number of recognised autoimmune or collagen diseases, in association with a remote carcinoma, or by itself. Typically, there is progressive muscle weakness, with muscle pain and tenderness, associated with systemic ill-health. Serum muscle enzymes (for example, creatine kinase) are increased, indicating muscle breakdown, and the ESR may be raised. Electromyography reveals evidence of a combination of primary muscle disease with signs of denervation. Muscle biopsy shows necrosis of muscle fibres associated with inflammatory infiltrate.

Immunosuppressive drug therapy (prednisolone, azathioprine, methotrexate or cyclophosphamide) and plasmapheresis are the present mainstays of treatment of inflammatory muscle diseases. Resolution of symptoms with increased muscle strength can be expected in those with acute polymyositis, but the response to treatment in patients with chronic long-standing muscle weakness (many of whom have only mildly elevated plasma muscle enzyme concentrations and a normal ESR) is less satisfactory. The success of treatment is monitored by the return of muscle strength and, less reliably, by falling serum muscle enzymes.

High-dose prednisolone (60–120 mg daily) is generally considered to be the first line of treatment. Many patients show a rapid and satisfactory improvement, so that steroid dosage can be lowered and adjusted to alternate-day therapy, reducing to a maintenance regime of prednisolone in doses of about 15–30 mg on alternate days.

Azathioprine and other cytotoxic drugs may be held in reserve for cases in which prednisolone treatment is unsuccessful. However, many would introduce azathioprine (75–100 mg daily) with prednisolone (60–100 mg on alternate days) from the beginning, in order to reduce the side effects of high-dose steroid treatment. In particular, high-dose steroids themselves may induce muscle atrophy thereby compounding the original problem. More potent cytotoxics, such as cyclophosphamide, probably are best held in reserve for those unresponsive to azathioprine and prednisolone. Plasma exchange (volume up to 5%–6% of body weight exchanged per week in up to ten exchanges, each plasmapheresis followed by human serum immune globulin 10 g) may also be employed in cases unresponsive to prednisolone and azathioprine.

Muscle Cramps

Painful muscle cramps are common but ill-understood. Muscle pain and cramps on exercise may be symptomatic of McArdle's disease (muscle phosphorylase deficiency) or other metabolic muscle disorder, but frequently no cause is found. In McArdle's disease, the inherited absence of glycogen phosphorylase leads to failure of breakdown of muscle glycogen. This is associated with a rise in blood lactate or pyruvate after exercise. It can be relieved by large doses of glucose, by insulin which facilitates glucose uptake, or by glucagon or adrenaline which act on the liver to raise blood glucose levels.

Muscle cramps are common in those who are dehydrated or salt-depleted. They are also a frequent complaint in pregnancy. Most common of all are the benign but distressing nocturnal cramps experienced by many otherwise normal people. Quinine is the traditional remedy.

Quinine

Quinine, along with phenytoin and calcium, may relieve muscle spasms by membrane stabilisation. Other membrane stabilisers, all of which prevent conduction of the action potential without altering the level of the resting membrane potential, include local anaesthetics as well as a number of fish toxins, for example the puffer fish in the Pacific and butter clams in Alaska. Membrane stabilisers may also relieve myotonia, but with the exception of phenytoin, usually do not affect myokymia.

Quinine (sulphate, bisulphate, hydrochloride and other salts) is a natural antimalarial obtained from the bark of *Cinchona* species, originally found in the Chilean Andes and brought to Europe by Jesuits in the seventeenth century. Quinine stabilises nerve terminals and skeletal muscle fibre membranes, and inhibits the response to acetylcholine. It is a basic drug with a pK_a of 8.4. The percentage of drug administered that is absorbed varies from 0% at pH 1 to 18% at pH 8. Quinine is widely distributed in the body, does not accumulate and is hydroxylated in the liver with urinary excretion of metabolites. Since the plasma half-life is short, quinine should be given 6- to 8-hourly.

Cinchonism with tinnitus, impaired hearing, blurring of vision, nausea and headache, skin sensitivity and inhibition of the synthesis of vitamin K-dependent clotting factors, usually results only from high-dose treatment of malaria. Retinal toxicity, however, may be idiosyncratic as well as dose-related, with retinal vascular spasm, loss of colour vision and sometimes loss of sight. Toxic effects on the heart are only observed when quinine is given intravenously, with a fall in blood pressure, depression of the R segment, and reduction or abolition of the T wave.

Quinine augments the effects of neuromuscular blocking agents, and should not be used acutely with suxamethonium. Severe painful muscle cramps as a result of dialysis, usually when the dialysate contains a low concentration of sodium, or when suxamethonium triggers an attack of acute discomfort followed by paraesthesia, improve with quinine as does the cramp of idiopathic recurrent rhabdomyolysis accompanying muscle breakdown after exercise.

Acute Inflammatory Polyneuropathy

Typically, the patient with an acute inflammatory polyneuropathy, or Guillain–Barré syndrome, presents with subacute weakness affecting particularly the proximal muscles of the arms and legs to begin with, associated with distal paraesthesiae. Weakness and sensory loss progress over a period of about 3 weeks, but then plateau and begin to recover. Recovery takes many months and may be incomplete, particularly in the elderly. Some patients can identify a preceding viral or nonspecific illness some weeks prior to the onset of their neuropathy. There are striking similarities between acute inflammatory polyneuropathy in humans and experimental allergic neuritis in animals. The latter is the result of an autoimmune response to immunisation with nerve antigens, and it is presumed that a similar mechanism is responsible for the analogous disease in humans. Such observations have led to the use of prednisolone and other immunosuppressants, as well as plasmapheresis, in the treatment of acute inflammatory polyneuropathy. However, the tendency for the disease to remit spontaneously has made it difficult to establish unequivocally whether any such treatment is of real value. Indeed, recent carefully controlled clinical trials have suggested that prednisolone, rather than being of benefit, may actually be associated with increased residual disability. The situation with plasmapheresis is more encouraging. Similarly well-controlled trials have indicated that plasmapheresis can increase the rate of recovery in selected patients.

An added difficulty is that some patients with what appears to start as a typical acute inflammatory polyneuropathy do not recover spontaneously, but continue to progress. If motor weakness and sensory loss continue to get worse for more than 6 weeks after the onset, it is likely that one is dealing not with an acute inflammatory polyneuropathy, but with what is called a chronic demyelinating neuropathy. Chronic demyelinating neuropathies are steroid-responsive, and commonly relapse when steroid dosage is reduced or the drugs are withdrawn, hence they are termed chronic relapsing demyelinating neuropathies.

In a proportion of patients with acute inflammatory polyneuropathy, motor weakness progresses rapidly to involve respiratory and bulbar muscles, requiring ventilatory support. In addition, the autonomic nervous system is often involved leading to tachycardia, arrhythmias and even cardiac arrest. Thus, this condition still carries a substantial mortality. Against this background, the relative risks and benefits of treatment must be balanced against the problems of ventilatory failure, autonomic disturbance and chronic residual fixed deficit in those who recover.

A general plan of management first focuses attention upon monitoring respiratory function and swallowing. A useful clinical clue to those at risk of ventilatory failure is the involvement of the facial or bulbar muscles. In those with mild disease, steroids and plasmapheresis can probably be withheld. In those with severe progressive disease, and especially in those with signs of imminent ventilatory failure, plasmapheresis should be instituted. Steroids probably should be withheld unless there is evidence of continued progression 6 weeks after the onset of the disease.

Motor Neurone Disease

Progressive degeneration of the corticomotoneurone pathway and anterior horn cells leads to combination of signs of an upper motoneurone lesion (muscle weakness, spasticity, brisk tendon reflexes and extensor plantar responses) with those of damage to the lower motoneurone (muscle weakness with wasting, and fasciculation). The disease may be most evident in anterior horn cells innervating the limbs (progressive muscular atrophy), or bulbar muscles (bulbar palsy), or may affect both upper and lower motoneurones innervating limbs (amyotrophic lateral sclerosis) or bulbar muscles (mixed pseudo- and bulbar palsy). Higher mental function and sensation generally are spared, as are the sphincters. Unfortunately, no treatment alters the course of motor neurone disease, and there are no definite clues as to its cause.

Up to two-thirds of patients with amyotrophic lateral sclerosis have a decremental response to nerve stimulation, which can be improved by anticholinesterases. Drugs such as neostigmine may produce a little improvement in muscle weakness for a short period of time. Muscle cramps may be helped by quinine sulphate or phenytoin. Spasticity may be improved by diazepam or baclofen. Control of dribbling, speech and swallowing may be improved temporarily by anticholinergics. Dysphagia may require the operation of cricopharyngeal myotomy. Intelligent use of mechanical aids, including devices to help communication, may be of considerable value.

Recently, attention has focused on thyroid-releasing hormone (TRH; L-pyroglutamyl-L-histidyl-L-prolinamide). TRH nerve endings are anatomically located around motor nuclei in the brain stem and spinal cord and TRH has been found to augment spinal reflexes in animals. Levels of TRH in the CSF of patients with motor neurone disease have been found to be reduced. Systemic administration of TRH, in very large doses, has been claimed to produce a transient increase in muscle strength in motor neurone disease. However, this has not proved to be a reliable practical means of therapy, although it has led to the development of longer-acting analogues of TRH which are now under clinical trial.

Further Reading

Albuquerque EX, Eldefrawi AT (eds) (1983) Myasthenia gravis. Chapman and Hall, London

10 Treatment of Disorders Involving the Autonomic Nervous System

Autonomic Failure

Autonomic failure occurs as a result of preganglionic or postganglionic autonomic neuropathy, or where there is an extensive defect in the central segment of autonomic reflexes, as in tetraplegia, or (rarely) in failure of the sensory limb of the buffer reflexes. Different diseases affect different parts of the autonomic system, resulting in different patterns of autonomic failure. Autonomic defects that are asymptomatic and detectable only by tests are not usually worth treating.

Causes of Symptomatic Autonomic Failure

Progressive Autonomic Failure

This can be progressive over many years, without any other neurological lesion. Often, the sympathetic lesion is mainly postganglionic, and precedes parasympathetic failure. Cause unknown.

Progressive Autonomic Failure with Olivopontocerebellar Atrophy or Striatonigral Degeneration (Multisystem Atrophy)

As well as autonomic failure, there is clinical evidence of striatonigral degeneration or olivopontocerebellar atrophy, with parkinsonian features, ataxia or dysarthria. The parkinsonism often comprises mainly rigidity and akinesia, rather than tremor. Occasionally, multisystem atrophy (MSA) is familial. The sympathetic lesion tends to be largely preganglionic. Cause unknown.

Diabetic Autonomic Failure

Symptomatic autonomic failure occurs only in insulin-dependent diabetics. Diabetes does not have to be very long-standing, but many poorly controlled diabetics do not develop it. The parasympathetic system is usually involved first, sympathetic functions being preserved until a late stage.

Tetraplegia and High Paraplegia

The cranial parasympathetic is intact, and connected to the baroreceptor afferents. The sacral parasympathetic and the sympathetic are decentralised. However, they are not inactive, and vasomotor and sudomotor discharges can be provoked by local stimuli. These responses may be inappropriate (autonomic dysreflexia). Inappropriate vasoconstriction can cause paroxysmal hypertension, particularly if the cord lesion is above the level of the sympathetic splanchnic outflow (about T-6), leaving the splanchnic outflow under the control of the isolated cord. Inappropriate sweating when body temperature is not raised can cause hypothermia. Similarly, the isolated sacral parasympathetic functions autonomously after a period of spinal shock. If there is extensive cord infarction, on the other hand, there may be preganglionic denervation due to loss of the intermediolateral cell column.

Familial Dysautonomia (Riley–Day Syndrome)

This autosomal recessive disease of Ashkenazi Jews, with afferent and preganglionic autonomic cell loss, as well as a generalised neuropathy, and a characteristic facial appearance is characterised by an outstanding ability for breathholding (with carotid body denervation).

Amyloidosis

Here, autonomic failure is believed to be due to local infiltration, with amyloid deposits in the spinal roots or the myenteric plexus. The rectal wall is usually involved. Occasionally there is amyloid infiltration of the baroreflex afferent fibres, causing labile hypertension.

Carcinomatous Autonomic Neuropathy

Sometimes, but not always, there is evidence of a generalised neuropathy as well.

Alcohol

Symptoms of orthostatic hypotension are rare in uncomplicated alcoholic peripheral neuropathy unless very severe, although tests of autonomic function may be abnormal at an earlier stage. In this respect alcoholic neuropathy resembles other dying-back neuropathies, where autonomic symptoms occur late.

Acute Autonomic Neuropathy

This is probably a form of Guillain–Barré syndrome, in which the autonomic system is selectively involved. Antibodies against autonomic cholinergic fibres have been demonstrated. Recovery may be complete or incomplete, and can take years. Acute or subacute autonomic failure in association with the full Guillain-Barré picture is also well described and can be severe. Patients who are paralysed by their somatic neuropathy may become hypotensive if propped up in bed, and can suffer brain damage as a result.

Drugs

Peripheral neuropathy associated with vincristine toxicity often has an autonomic preponderance. Symptoms suggesting autonomic neuropathy have been described in heavy metal poisoning (thallium, arsenic, mercury), and occasionally following treatment of angina with perhexiline maleate.

Many drugs can cause (reversible) autonomic symptoms, particularly orthostatic hypotension, owing to their main pharmacological actions. These include vasodilators (prazosin, hydralazine), centrally acting hypotensives (methyldopa, clonidine), ganglion-blocking drugs (hexamethonium, mecamylamine), adrenergic neuron blockers (guanethidine, debrisoquine, bethanidine), α-adrenergic antagonists (phenoxybenzamine, phentolamine, labetalol) and angiotensin-converting enzyme inhibitors (captopril). Other groups of drugs cause these symptoms less often (phenothiazines, barbiturates, some tricyclics, monoamine oxidase inhibitors). These effects are reversible and dose-related.

Other Congenital Diseases with Neuropathy

Autonomic symptoms may occur in porphyria, peroneal muscular atrophy, Friedreich's ataxia and congenital sensory neuropathy.

Other Diseases

Autonomic features are sometimes conspicuous in chronic renal failure, rheumatoid arthritis, Chagas' disease and leprosy.

Tests of Autonomic Function

Sympathetic Function

Blood Pressure Response to Standing Up from a Lying Position

Normal response: systolic BP approximately unchanged; diastolic often rises a little.
Abnormal response: systolic BP falls more than 30 mmHg.
Doubtful response: systolic BP falls 10–30 mmHg.

This tests the overall function of the baroreflex pathway. It does not distinguish afferent, central and efferent lesions. It is normal in patients with active (vasovagal) faints, where fainting is caused by reflex vasodilatation accompanied by vagal slowing.

Blood Pressure Response to Stresses

This includes responses to such stresses as: sudden unexpected noise, mental arithmetic, submaximal handgrip sustained for 90 s, hand immersed in icy water for 90 s.

Normal response: diastolic BP rises at least 10 mmHg.
Abnormal response: no rise.
Doubtful response: rise of less than 10 mmHg.

This response is not dependent on baroreceptor afferent or baroreflex central excitability, but tests the integrity of the sympathetic outflow. There is a large proportion of doubtful responses in normal people.

Sweat Test

Heat the patient (sun lamp and hot tea) after dusting the skin with a sweat indicator powder (e.g. quinarizin). This tests the cholinergic sympathetic sudomotor pathway. It has the advantage that it can detect a patchy, partial or asymmetric loss. The response is centrally generated, so intact sensory nerves are not required.

Infusion of Noradrenaline and Tyramine

An increased response to noradrenaline (NA) and loss of response to tyramine indicates a postganglionic lesion. Some increase in the response to both indicates a preganglionic lesion. If the lesion is mixed the results may be confusing. The test is not very safe, as adrenergic denervation hypersensitivity of the heart can make it liable to arrhythmias.

Parasympathetic Function

Valsalva Manoeuvre

Maintain an expiratory pressure of 40 mmHg for 15 s, then breathe normally. Blowing up a sphygmomanometer will do. It is best to provide a small side hole in the mouth tube, so as to prevent cheating. The physiology of the events in this manoeuvre is complex, but the bradycardia that follows the increased pulse volume of the early postexpiratory phase is a vagal baroreflex effect.

Normal response: normal postexpiratory rebound of heart rate and BP.
Abnormal response: loss of postexpiratory bradycardia.

Pulse Rate Response to Standing Up

There is an immediate tachycardia followed by a reflex bradycardia maximal after about 30 beats. Measure the 15th and 30th R–R intervals on ECG.

Normal response: 30:15 ratio more than 1.04:1.
Abnormal response: 30:15 ratio less than 1.

Symptomatic Treatment of Autonomic Failure
(Table 10.1)

Cardiovascular System

The most prominent symptoms of autonomic failure here manifest themselves by a loss of BP regulation, which can occur through various mechanisms. Several segments of the circulation vary their resistance according to fluctuations in their local blood flow need.
For example:

Cerebral. Resistance varies so as to maintain flow constant in the face of BP fluctuations. Resistance varies so as to increase flow if pCO_2 rises, or if pH or pO_2 falls.
Muscle. Resistance varies so as to increase muscle blood flow when the muscle is exercised.

Gut. Resistance varies so as to increase flow postprandially.
Skin. Flow is increased if skin temperature is high, reduced if low.

None of these local responses requires an intact autonomic system. Each of these major organs uses a large proportion of the cardiac output. So if one sector varies its requirement and BP is to be kept constant, something must change to compensate; either the resistance of other sectors of the circulation, or the cardiac output must change, or both. These compensatory changes involve autonomic reflex control of peripheral resistance and cardiac output. Thus for example there is reflex vasoconstriction of skin and gut when vigorous muscle activity occurs or is likely. If these compensations are less than perfect, then the resulting change in BP will bring in the high-pressure baroreceptor reflex to adjust BP.

In addition, the baroreflex operates to compensate for changes in posture. On standing up, not only does the height of the head above the heart increase, but venous return to the heart is considerably reduced, since about 700 ml blood leaves the chest and pools in the abdomen and legs. Carotid baroceptor reflexes are believed to act largely on the splanchnic resistance. If the baroreflex fails, the BP becomes unstable, with orthostatic hypotension, recumbent hypertension, exercise hypotension, postprandial hypotension and hypersensitivity of BP to drugs. Changes in atrial pressure also affect atrial low-pressure receptors, which reflexly act both on peripheral resistance (mainly muscle resistance) and also on the renin–angiotensin system so as to alter blood volume in the compensatory direction. Loss of this reflex results in recumbent polyuria and Na^+ loss, and orthostatic circulatory overload with ankle oedema.

Although the resistance of the cerebral circulation is self-regulating, so as to maintain a constant flow, its response is not instantaneous. A patient with loss of buffer reflexes who has recumbent hypertension and orthostatic hypotension may faint on standing even though the BP does not drop to the normal limit of autoregulation, if the cerebral resistance cannot follow the changes called for quickly enough.

The response to adrenergic drugs is particularly exaggerated where there is not only loss of the buffer reflexes, but also cardiac and vasomotor adrenergic receptor supersensitivity. Such supersensitivity is much greater where the denervation is postganglionic than where it is preganglionic. Adrenergic drugs are of little use in autonomic failure, as they cause increased recumbent hypertension and do not prevent orthostatic hypotension. The response is supersensitive and hard to control. No drug will compensate for the loss of buffer reflexes, but the effects are minimised by preventing the recumbent polyuria and Na^+ loss which result in loss of circulating volume.

Practical points in the treatment of circulatory symptoms in autonomic failure:

1. Only treat if symptomatic.
2. Do not aggravate recumbent hypertension.
3. Aim to control blood volume, and reduce pooling.

4. Improved mobility is beneficial, since it discourages recumbent sodium loss.

The methods available are:

1. Tilt head up at night, to activate the renin–angiotensin system, and discourage recumbent sodium loss. Measure urinary sodium and potassium output and balance, haematocrit, plasma proteins, urea and electrolytes and weight.

2. Fludrocortisone (0.05–0.3 mg/day p.o.) has at least two effects. First, it increases blood volume by promoting sodium retention. Second, even in a dose inadequate to alter blood volume it can increase the effect of endogenous NA release without causing recumbent hypertension (i.e. it can partially restore the gain of the sympathetic component of the buffer reflex), possibly by increasing adrenergic receptor population.

3. External support by elastic stockings or G suit has the effect of reducing the haemodynamic adjustment necessary between the recumbent and upright postures, so reducing both recumbent hypertension and orthostatic hypotension for as long as the aid is worn. It does not prevent recumbent hypovolaemia, so on removing the G suit the patient may be worse off than ever.

4. Pressor drugs are not useful in general. Although they will reduce orthostatic hypotension they may aggravate recumbent hypertension dangerously, particularly where there is a postganglionic component, and receptor supersensitivity. When the lesion is preganglionic, tyramine plus MAOI will have a similar effect.

5. Dihydroergotamine has been shown to have an α-agonist effect on capacitance vessels, and works well by i.v. infusion (but plasma half-life is only 0.5 h). Absorption is too erratic for oral treatment to be reliable, and long-term infusion is not yet practicable. It reduces the compliance of the capacitance vessels, and hence reduces pooling and loss of venous return on standing. No reliably absorbed oral drug acting primarily on capacitance vessels is yet available.

6. Indomethacin (50–200 mg/day p.o.), or flurbiprofen (150–200 mg/day p.o.) have been used in divided doses, on the grounds that they are prostaglandin synthetase inhibitors, and some prostaglandins are vasodilators. Alternatively, indomethacin may potentiate endogenous NA and angiotensin by its effect on presynaptic prostaglandin and angiotensin receptors on adrenergic nerves (i.e. by increasing the gain of the failing buffer reflex output pathway).

7. Clonidine has no antihypertensive effect in autonomic failure, since that effect is exerted on the vasomotor centre, but its peripheral α-agonist effect is then revealed. Under these circumstances, like other α-adrenergic drugs, it will cause an increase in recumbent hypertension.

8. Other drug combinations that could be theoretically appropriate would be those which amplified the residual α-adrenergic vasomotor activity, by

prolonging adrenergic action and promoting spread to nearby supersensitive denervated receptors, either by inhibiting presynaptic NA reuptake (secondary amine tricyclic drugs such as desipramine), or by inhibiting postsynaptic NA breakdown.

9. In autonomic failure with parkinsonism (MSA), levodopa treatment may aggravate postural hypotension by a central effect. In any case, levodopa is usually relatively ineffective for the movement disorder in MSA, and striatal binding affinity for dopamine is reduced. Bromocriptine (2.5–30 mg/day p.o., p.c., building up slowly), a direct-acting postsynaptic dopamine agonist, may improve parkinsonism, but often causes postural hypotension.

10. Loss of exercise tolerance occurs as a result of at least two factors. First, cardiac output fails to respond adequately to exercise, the only increase being due to the (Starling's law) response to increased venous return. Second, exercise-induced muscle vasodilation is not compensated for by vasoconstriction elsewhere (gut, skin), so that exercise-induced syncope occurs. This is made worse when there are other stimuli causing locally controlled vasodilation elsewhere (postprandial, hot weather).

Exercise syncope is more likely to occur early in progressive autonomic failure or multisystem atrophy, where the lesion is mainly sympathetic, than in diabetic autonomic failure, where the initial lesion is mainly parasympathetic, resulting, for example, in a high fixed heart rate.

Drug treatment of exercise syncope is not satisfactory. β-Adrenergic drugs would be expected to benefit exercise syncope by increasing cardiac output, but at the cost of some recumbent hypertension. The main danger with them however is that in autonomic failure the denervated heart may be supersensitive to them, and liable to serious arrhythmias. Even without adrenergic drugs, sudden death due to cardiac arrhythmias is common in autonomic failure.

Postural Symptoms and Autonomic Dysreflexia in Tetraplegia

In tetraplegia, the cardiovascular autonomic problems are different from those seen in autonomic neuropathy. Postural symptoms are caused by disconnection of the sympathetic efferent pathway, while the vagal control of the heart is intact. There is no marked adrenergic receptor denervation supersensitivity, although there is some increased sensitivity to infused NA, because of the loss of buffer reflexes. Even if there is extensive cord infarction below the level of the lesion, resulting in intermediolateral cell loss, the denervation is preganglionic and supersensitivity is not marked. If the sympathetic cell column is intact, however, and it usually is, then autonomic dysreflexia may occur, provoked by painful stimuli below the lesion, flexor or extensor muscle spasms, a full bladder or bowel, reflex erection or ejaculation. Autonomic dysreflexia can produce severe paroxysmal hypertension, aggravated by the loss of buffer reflexes. Autonomic dysreflexia can be minimised by attention to bladder and bowel, and antispastic and antispasm drugs such as baclofen or diazepam, so as to reduce the stimulus to the cord.

The lack of baroreflexes and of adrenergic drive to the heart in tetraplegia can result in exaggerated bradycardia and hypotension in response to vagal stimuli such as tracheal suction.

Gastrointestinal Tract

Diarrhoea in autonomic failure is often nocturnal, intermittent and watery, with incontinence (sphincter denervation). It may be related to stasis and bacterial deconjugation of bile acids. Its occurrence at night or during sleep may result from the additional effect of sleep atonia on an already compromised bowel and sphincter. After excluding steatorrhoea (faecal fat, barium meal, jejunal biopsy), codeine (10–60 mg/day p.o.) or tetracycline (250–750 mg/day p.o.) are usually effective. Gastroparesis due to parasympathetic denervation may cause troublesome vomiting. Metoclopramide (20–30 mg/day p.o.) or domperidone (30–40 mg/day p.o.) are effective.

Genitourinary Tract

The bladder is affected both by sensory loss and parasympathetic detrusor denervation, causing an atonic bladder with chronic retention, overflow incontinence, a large residual volume and hesitancy of micturition. In these circumstances it is necessary to exclude obstruction at bladder neck or prostate level (cytoscopy, intravenous pyelography, urodynamics). The bladder neck may be weak, in which case voiding by abdominal straining or suprapubic pressure may be effective, particularly in women. If it is not weak then bladder neck resection may be needed. Voiding contractions may be improved with bethanechol. If there is still gross retention, a catheter may be needed.

An uninhibited bladder (due to loss of the β-adrenergic inhibitory innervation of detrusor) is a rare occurrence in progressive autonomic failure, but it is common in MSA, because of the associated central lesions. In MSA, impotence, urgency incontinence, poor stream and loss of sphincter tone can all occur. The bladder neck is incompetent and there is denervation of the striated anal and urethral sphincters, with associated cell loss in Onuf's nucleus in the lower sacral cord segments. There is thought to be loss of basal ganglia inhibition of the pontine micturition centre. At a later stage, the intermediolateral cell columns and cells in the pontine micturition centre degenerate as well, so there is superadded retention and loss of micturition reflexes.

Loss of erectile potency, and failure of ejaculation or retrograde ejaculation are common in autonomic failure. Although there exist both lumbar sympathetic and sacral parasympathetic pathways (both probably VIP-ergic) serving erection, it is not clear that the sacral parasympathetic pathway is present in all men. Retrograde ejaculation, caused by failure of contraction of the α-adrenergically innervated bladder neck, can sometimes be relieved with desipramine (50–100 mg, 1–2 h before ejaculation) which potentiates NA by reuptake inhibition.

Erectile impotence can be treated with a penile implant. Alternatively, erectile impotence (either primary or associated with autonomic failure) can be temporarily overcome with intracavernosal phenoxybenzamine (5 mg) or papaverine (40 mg), which causes erection lasting 1–4 h.

Respiratory System

In patients with autonomic failure, respiratory arrest may be precipitated by anaesthesia, drugs or pneumonia. Sleep apnoea in autonomic failure is often due to both central and peripheral mechanisms with loss of central respiratory output during sleep, loss of reflex respiratory mechanisms, and laryngeal (abductor palsy) obstruction, as well as oropharyngeal collapse during sleep. In addition, the motor output to the respiratory muscles may be interrupted by high cord lesions.

Thermoregulation

Loss of sweating results in a reduced capacity for regulation against temperature rise, and liability to heat stroke. In heat stroke the BP can fall (heating of the brain stem causes loss of vasomotor control), so orthostatic hypotension is made worse. In spinal cord lesions, thermoregulatory responses, like vasomotor responses, can be inappropriate below the lesion, with inappropriate sweating and shivering-like spasms. The effect of this is most marked where the lesion is above the thoracolumbar outflow, so that in lesions above T-1 even sudomotor control of the head and face is decentralised. Behavioural thermoregulatory control has to take over from autonomic. Shivering is centrally generated, and is preserved in autonomic failure of whatever cause, unless there is involvement of somatic motor pathways, as in high cord lesions or the Guillain–Barré syndrome.

The Bladder in Neurological Disease

Patterns of Neurological Bladder Disorder

The pattern of bladder disorder in neurological diseases does vary with the site of the lesion, as there is a hierarchy in the control of the bladder, just as there is hierarchical control in the motor system.

Table 10.1. Aspects of autonomic failure that may require treatment

System involved	Consequences
Cardiovascular system	Loss of baroreflexes, causing orthostatic hypotension or recumbent hypertension Loss of cardiovascular response to exercise Postprandial hypotension Recumbent polyuria and Na^+ loss Receptor denervation supersensitivity Autonomic dysreflexia (tetraplegia, high paraplegia and clonidine withdrawal) Arteriovenous shunting in the periphery
Gastrointestinal tract	Diarrhoea Gastroparesis and vomiting Megaviscus disorders Ulceration
Genitourinary tract	Atonic bladder Uninhibited bladder Loss of erectile potency Ejaculatory failure (either retrograde or complete)
Respiratory system	Respiratory arrests Sleep apnoea
Thermoregulation	Loss of sweating Nocturnal or gustatory sweating Hypothermia Heat stroke
Extremities	Cutaneous vasoconstriction due to adrenergic supersensitivity Increased peripheral blood flow with osteoporosis and arteriovenous shunting Loss of regulation of peripheral flow

Cerebral Lesions (the "Cerebral Bladder")

Cerebral lesions, particularly parasagittal lesions, may increase or decrease the normal inhibition of the urge to void (depending on the site of the lesion), so that urgency incontinence or alternatively retention with loss of the urge to void can occur. Detrusor inhibition and increase in striated and smooth muscle sphincter tone (the accommodation reaction) is a normal reflex function which occurs during the filling phase as a response to increasing bladder volume. Accommodation has reciprocal inhibition with the reflexes that initiate and maintain the voiding act. The accommodation reflex is impaired, and urgency incontinence promoted, by lesions in the superior frontal gyrus or the adjacent anterior cingulate gyrus, while more posterior lesions (paracentral lobule) can result in sphincter overactivity and retention. However, coordination of the parts of the voiding act itself is preserved in cerebral lesions, since the spinal segmental mechanisms remain connected to the pontine micturition centre.

Spinal Lesions (the "Spinal Bladder")

The effect of a spinal lesion, isolating the bladder from the pontine micturition centre of Barrington, is seen in its purest form in paraplegia and tetraplegia. Even so, the bladder may vary from atonic (in chronic retention with overflow incontinence), through the reflex bladder (triggered by segmental stimuli such as abdominal percussion), to the irritable bladder with uninhibited detrusor contractions occurring at small volume. Poorly sustained detrusor contractions and detrusor–sphincter dyssynergia (loss of reciprocal inhibition between detrusor and the striated sphincter) are features of the spinal bladder.

Cauda Equina Lesions (the "Cauda Equina Bladder")

In cauda equina lesions, due for example to low spinal injury, myelomeningocele or central lumbar disc protrusion, the bladder is generally atonic with chronic urinary retention, although coordinated detrusor response to filling is sometimes seen. There is denervation of the striated sphincters, and a preganglionic parasympathetic neuropathy. The sympathetic supply is intact.

Autonomic Neuropathy (the "Neuropathic Bladder")

In autonomic neuropathy the situation is more complex, and depends on the cause of autonomic failure (q.v.). Besides sympathetic and parasympathetic denervation (degeneration of the intermediolateral cell column), there may be degeneration in long tracts, causing detrusor–sphincter dyssynergia and uninhibited detrusor contractions. There may also be denervation of the striated sphincter, aggravating the incontinence, particularly in the Shy–Drager syndrome.

Urgent attempts should be made to treat chronic retention and incontinence in patients with neurological disease as, besides the misery of incontinence, ureteric reflux and chronic or recurrent urinary tract infection occur, and often result in progressive renal damage. This is most clearly seen in traumatic paraplegia, where chronic renal failure due to pyelonephritis and hydronephrosis is still a common cause of death.

Methods for Treating the Neurological Bladder

1. Drugs (Table 10.2)

Innervation of the detrusor is parasympathetic cholinergic muscarinic, while innervation of the bladder neck smooth muscle is at least in part sympathetic

Table 10.2. Drugs acting therapeutically on the bladder[a]

Action	Detrusor	Bladder neck	Striated sphincter
Inhibit	Propantheline (15–60 mg/day)	Phenoxybenzamine (10–20 mg/day)	Baclofen (10–60 mg/day)
	Emepronium (200–600 mg/day)	Alfuzosin[c] (10–30 mg/day)	Diazepam (2–30 mg/day)
	Imipramine[b] (25–150 mg/day)		Dantrolene (25–600 mg/day)
	Isoprenaline (20–60 mg/day)		
Stimulate	Carbachol (2–6 mg/day)	Orciprenaline (20–80 mg/day)	Neostigmine (45–150 mg/day)
	Bethanechol (30–120 mg/day)	Phenylpropanolamine (15–30 mg/day)	
	Distigmine (5–20 mg/day)	Ephedrine (30–120 mg/day)	
		Imipramine[d] (25–150 mg/day)	

[a] Average total oral daily dosages
[b] Anticholinergic effect
[c] Selective α_1-adrenergic blocking drug, on trial at the time of writing
[d] α-Adrenergic effect (NA reuptake blockade)

α-adrenergic. α-Adrenergic blockade results in about 80% loss of urethral closure pressure. There is a β-adrenergic innervation of the bladder dome, which inhibits detrusor contraction, probably as part of the accommodation reflex.

Drugs are available which increase or decrease detrusor contractility, which increase or decrease urethral resistance and which reduce pelvic floor spasticity (Table 10.2). In order for any of these actions to be effective in promoting controlled and complete voiding, it is essential that the patient should retain some control over the filling and voiding phases of bladder function. A patient who has uninhibited and ill-sustained detrusor contractions with dyssynergia, causing incontinence with a large residual volume, is unlikely to be benefited by any drug. Drugs can alter the bladder's capacity and its tendency to initiate and sustain voiding contractions, but the time of administration in relation to the desired effect may be critical, and difficult to achieve in practice.

Neurological chronic retention can be treated by a drug increasing detrusor contractility, or by one reducing urethral resistance; but urodynamic investigation is needed first to see which site is at fault. Urgency incontinence with uninhibited detrusor contractions can be treated with drugs reducing detrusor contractility, while stress incontinence with loss of adequate urethral closure pressure is treated with drugs increasing urethral pressure, and from these may be chosen appropriately either a drug increasing tone in the bladder neck (e.g. ephedrine), or one increasing urethral turgor (oestrogen).

Drugs Increasing Detrusor Contractility

These may be used in chronic retention provided there is no urgency incontinence as well, and no outflow obstruction, either structural (e.g. prostate) or functional (dyssynergia).

Bethanechol is a parasympathomimetic, facilitating transmission through the pelvic ganglia as well as neuromuscular transmission at the detrusor. It is said to show some selectivity for these sites over other cholinergic synapses, but side effects such as abdominal cramps, vomiting and diarrhoea, bradycardia and hypotension do occur.

Carbachol is an analogue of acetylcholine, resistant to acetylcholinesterase, with a prolonged action at muscarinic and nicotinic synapses. Its side effects are similar to those of bethanechol, in spite of its different mode of action, but can be more severe.

Neostigmine and pyridostigmine, being anticholinesterase drugs, do have an action in increasing detrusor contractility, but they are nonselective, with gastrointestinal and cardiovascular side effects, such as bradycardia and colic.

Distigmine is a long-acting anticholinesterase sometimes given for atonic bladder, but it is nonselective and expensive.

Anticholinesterases and carbachol, besides acting directly at the parasympathetic terminals on detrusor, also act at the cholinergic autonomic ganglia, both sympathetic and parasympathetic. The action at parasympathetic ganglia in this context does no harm, but activation of sympathetic ganglia may need to be counteracted by peripheral blockade. Alpha-blockade would block the increased tone in the bladder neck, and beta-blockade would prevent the β-adrenergic inhibition of detrusor. There are no adrenergic blockers which are selective for these sites.

Drugs Reducing Detrusor Contractility

These are anticholinergic muscarinic competitive blockers. Propantheline and emepronium are quaternary ammonium compounds which do not enter the brain and therefore do not cause the central effects of atropine. Their peripheral effects are not selective for the bladder. In the usual dose they are far less effective on the detrusor than atropine, and the dose may need to be increased. The side effects include constipation, visual blurring (loss of accommodation) and tachycardia.

Imipramine has an anticholinergic action, but it also stimulates α-adrenergic receptors in the bladder neck and urethral smooth muscle, increasing resting tone there. It is thought also to have an anaesthetic effect in the bladder and urethra, reducing the likelihood of reflex voiding contractions.

Detrusor activity can be reduced by ganglion-blocking drugs such as mecamylamine. This is obtained at the expense of symptoms such as postural hypotension, because sympathetic and parasympathetic ganglia are blocked indiscriminately.

Drugs Decreasing Urethral Resistance

Contraction of smooth muscle in bladder neck and proximal urethra is largely an α-adrenergic action, so urethral resistance is reduced by α-adrenergic receptor blockers.

Phenoxybenzamine is a suitable long-acting alpha-blocker, but the dose has to be started at a low level and increased slowly, until an adequate response is obtained, or until side effects such as postural hypotension or tachycardia occur.

Phentolamine is a short-acting alpha-blocker that can be used during urodynamic testing to discover whether alpha-blockade will aid voiding.

Drugs Increasing Urethral Resistance

Alpha-stimulating drugs such as ephedrine and phenylpropanolamine increase urethral closure pressure by their action on periurethral smooth muscle. Ephedrine is often used in the treatment of nocturnal enuresis in children. Owing to its central actions it can cause irritability, loss of appetite, and insomnia or poor sleep, the latter no doubt increasing its efficacy in nocturnal enuresis. Phenylpropanolamine has a similar mode of action peripherally, but has fewer central effects. It has also been used successfully to treat retrograde ejaculation in men (caused by α-adrenergic insufficiency at the bladder neck), as has desipramine (which prolongs the action of NA by blocking its reuptake at the adrenergic terminal).

In postmenopausal women, oestrogen deficiency can result in atrophy of urethral tissue, loss of turgor and stress incontinence, which can be treated by oestrogen replacement (e.g. oestradiol 1 mg/day for 3 weeks in every 4), alone or combined with progesterone, if there are none of the usual contraindications (thromboembolic disease, hypertension, migraine, hormone-dependent carcinoma, hepatic or renal disease).

Drugs Reducing Autonomic Dysreflexia

With complete or nearly complete cord lesions above about T-6, visceral distension (including bladder fullness) can precipitate uncontrolled sympathetic discharge with sweating, colic and hypertension, as well as flexion reflexes. Autonomic dysreflexia is discouraged by improvements to bladder emptying, and can be partially blocked with α-adrenergic blockers such as phenoxybenzamine (see p. 175).

Drugs for the Treatment of External Sphincter Spasticity

Antispastic drugs such as diazepam, baclofen and dantrolene can reduce tone in the striated sphincter, and are used (particularly baclofen) in the treatment of detrusor–sphincter dyssynergia. The intramural striated sphincter, unlike the surrounding periurethral striated muscle, is normally tonically active.

Treatment of Urinary Tract Infection

The common causes of ascending urinary tract infection in neurological patients are chronic retention, ureteric reflux and indwelling catheter. Urinary infection should be treated with antibiotics when it is symptomatic, and often when it is not. It is often impracticable to eradicate asymptomatic infection when there is an indwelling catheter. Chronic retention due to poor detrusor contractions or functional urethral obstruction can be treated with drugs, a drainage operation or intermittent self-catheterisation. Ascending infection can result in progressive renal damage and is treated with a high fluid intake, frequent bladder emptying and an appropriate antibiotic (urine culture for sensitivities). Urinary infection can sometimes be prevented by urinary acidification with hexamine mandelate, provided the kidney remains capable of making acid urine.

Reflex Training

Bladder training in the patient with a spinal bladder, with the aim of achieving an effective automatic or reflexly emptying bladder, is practised in many good spinal injury centres, but rarely elsewhere, perhaps because it is time-consuming. The aim is to train the patient to empty the bladder reflexly when required. The effective stimulus to the voiding reflex varies, but abdominal percussion or compression is the most commonly successful. However, the detrusor contractions may be poorly sustained and are often accompanied by dyssynergic contraction of the external urethral sphincter. This can cause poor voiding, leading to bladder trabeculation and hypertrophy, ureteric reflux, chronic retention and urinary infection. External sphincterotomy and occasionally transurethral resection of the bladder neck therefore tend to be done early in association with bladder training, particularly in male paraplegics. In men with a cauda equina lesion, with an atonic bladder and denervated sphincter, voiding by abdominal compression without a detrusor contraction is often possible; and in women even without sphincter paralysis (or surgery).

Urinal Devices

An external condom urinal and drainage bag (external catheter) is the usual method for treating drug-resistant incontinence in men, such as that caused by spinal trauma, multiple sclerosis, cauda equina lesion or cerebral incontinence. The condom sheath draining to a leg bag has replaced the rigid collecting sheath. The condom may be taped or glued on, depending on design, and may last 1–3 days between changes. The bladder may empty spontaneously or in response to a manoeuvre to provoke reflex voiding. A penile clamp, released when voiding is required, carries obvious risks of pressure ulceration, penile swelling, and urethral stricture, and patients must be made well aware of the danger of leaving the clamp on too long or too tight. Continence clamps for the female, such as the Edwards pubovaginal spring or the Bonnar inflatable intravaginal device depend on good fitting, and again if pressure is excessive erosion of the urethra will occur, particularly if there is sensory loss in sacral segments. There is no effective equivalent for women of the condom urinal, and many women with intractable incontinence have to wear plastic pants and pads.

Intermittent Self-Catheterisation

Introduced by Lapides as an alternative to chronic indwelling catheter, intermittent clean (nonsterile) self-catheterisation aims to drain the bladder completely 2–3 times a day, improving bacterial washout and reducing the likelihood of infection growing in the residual urine. Some patients manage partial voidings in between catheterisations. It is impracticable if the patient's arms are weak or clumsy (particularly in women) or if the patient is demented. Bladder health is improved and long-term renal damage reduced, in comparison with chronic indwelling catheter. Full sterile intermittent catheterisation had been previously used in hospitals, but is not usually practicable at home.

Indwelling Catheter

The traditional method of managing neurological retention or incontinence since the First World War, it has been increasingly recognised as a source of recurrent or persistent urinary tract infection, periurethral abscess, prostatitis, stone formation and occasionally bladder carcinoma, and in men epididymitis, epididymo-orchitis, and abscess, diverticulum or fistula at the penoscrotal angle. Some complications such as encrustation and stone formation can be greatly reduced by silicone rubber catheters and regular bladder washout, the correct size of catheter (not too large) and avoiding angulation of the catheter. The balloon should be inflated only just enough to stop the catheter coming out. Most patients find an indwelling catheter depressing, even when it solves intractable incontinence.

Catheterisation Procedure

1. Septrin, two tablets twice daily for 2 days when the catheter is inserted or changed.
2. Maintenance on urinary antiseptics, e.g. hexamine hippurate 1 g twice daily, or hexamine mandelate 1 g four times daily.
3. If infection occurs with suprapubic pain or blocked catheter, rotating antibiotics; frequent aseptic catheter changes may be necessary.
4. The catheter should be changed every 4 weeks routinely.
5. Regular bladder washouts (chlorhexidine gluconate 1 in 5000).

Drainage Operations

Chronic retention with urgency or overflow incontinence is commonly due to structural obstruction, such as prostatic hypertrophy or urethral stricture. When these common conditions coexist with neurological lesions, they are dealt with by conventional surgery. When the cause is entirely neurological, and the obstruction wholly functional (increased sphincter tone, or failure of sphincter relaxation), either drugs or surgery may be appropriate.

An effective sphincterotomy does not necessarily cause incontinence, as either the bladder neck mechanism alone or the striated sphincter mechanisms alone can often maintain continence. Cystometry and urethral pressure profile will demonstrate whether the failure to relax on attempted voiding is the fault of the bladder neck or the striated sphincter, so that the appropriate operation is done. Sphincterotomy is the common operation, as sphincter dyssynergia is common, and antispastic drugs are not always successful. If both operations have to be radical to give adequate emptying, the result is permanent incontinence. This is often acceptable in men, who can wear an external urinal device, and the problem rarely arises in women because the striated sphincter mechanisms are weaker. Small sphincterotomies, which can be repeated if necessary, are usually sufficient to reduce residual volume and reverse hydronephrosis, and do not cause incontinence. The indications are: high residual volume, high voiding pressure, vesicoureteric reflux, or upper tract dilatation. If external sphincterotomy fails, or if there is a lower motor neurone lesion and loss of external sphincter pressure, then bladder neck resection is appropriate.

An incomplete low cord lesion (below L2) can cause a relatively atonic bladder, with normal sympathetic innervation of the bladder neck, and sometimes spasticity of the external sphincter. This combination too may require sphincterotomy.

Surgery for Incontinence and Reflux

Conventional incontinence surgery is not often applicable where incontinence is due to a neurological lesion, since the incontinence is usually due to loss of sphincter control rather than misplacement of the bladder neck. When the incontinence is due to uninhibited detrusor contractions, intrathecal phenol or a selective (S-3) sacral rhizotomy can make the bladder more flaccid. Other operations for instability include prolonged distension, subtrigonal phenol injection, and augmentation cystoplasty.

Operations to raise outflow resistance include periurethral polytetra-fluoroethylene injection, colposuspension and artificial sphincters. Artificial sphincter implants (which can be opened and closed by the patient) can overcome neurological stress incontinence due to sphincter failure. Associated urge incontinence or detrusor hyperreflexia can be treated with drugs. It is necessary first to rule out or treat severe detrusor hyperreflexia, severe reflux, bladderstones, contracted fibrotic bladder, and infravesical obstruction. The prostheses are expensive, but effective, although there is an incidence of complications such as infection of the implant. This can only be avoided by meticulous surgical technique. Previously troublesome complications like erosion of the urethra have been reduced by design improvements. These devices are also used for incontinence of urological cause.

Ureteric reflux is a common complication in the spinal bladder, and is liable to lead to progressive renal damage. It can be successfully treated surgically (for example by reimplantation of the ureters) provided infravesical obstruction is dealt with first; but it may disappear spontaneously when the obstruction is removed.

Artificial Voiding by Stimulator

Radio-linked implants stimulating the conus medullaris, sacral anterior roots, pelvic nerves and detrusor muscle have been developed in the last decade. Stimulation at any site other than the sacral anterior (motor) root is likely to be painful, except in complete cord lesions, when it still may provoke reflex spasms. Direct stimulation of the detrusor muscle is likely to lead to electrode breakage owing to repeated movement of the electrodes when the bladder contracts. Conus stimulation evokes various reflex effects, of which voiding is one. Sacral anterior root stimulator implants require a sacral laminectomy, but have been reported to give good complete voiding (and consequently usually continence as well) in a series of over 50 patients, with a follow-up of up to 8 years. Their usefulness in conditions other than spinal injury has not yet been assessed.

Artificial Continence by Stimulator

Various vaginal and anal stimulators have been used, aiming to overcome neurological incontinence. They may work by activating the external urethral sphincter directly or by stimulation of the nerves to it, or (more likely) by provoking reflex contraction of the pelvic floor, or by inhibiting detrusor contractions by stimulating afferent nerve fibres to the accommodation reflex. The last mechanism will work only in urgency incontinence. Vaginal stimulators in particular are effective in a proportion of cases. The accommodation reflex can be provoked in normal people by voluntary sphincter contraction as well as by bladder filling. It is not surprising then that it can also be provoked by perineal (anal or vaginal) stimulation, which itself provokes reflex sphincter closure. Electrical stimulation is more convenient than mechanical stimulation, and good results have been reported with electrical stimulators that have been shown not to activate the urethral sphincters directly.

Diversion Operations

Urinary diversions are considered only where there is intractable ureteric reflux, or total incontinence, particularly in women. The ureters are implanted usually into an ileal or colonic loop. The ureteric reflux is not necessarily cured, and ascending infection and progressive renal damage are usual in the long term, so diversion is to be avoided, particularly in patients with a long life expectancy. Reabsorption of urinary electrolytes does occur, particularly from ileal loops. Chronic infection of the remaining bladder (occurring because there is no drainage of it) may necessitate cystectomy.

The Bowel

Faecal compaction and chronic constipation are especially common in neurological diseases in bedridden, elderly, immobile patients, particularly in parkinsonism; and with anticholinergic drug or narcotic treatment or in the presence of dehydration.

Hydration, bran, prunes, withdrawal of anticholinergic drugs, and others with a similar action (e.g. antihistamines, tricyclic drugs, phenothiazines), and giving Fybogel (ispaghula husk; 1–2 sachets daily) or other fibrous preparations, and dioctyl sodium sulphosuccinate 100 mg three times daily, all relieve constipation, although manual removal, suppositories or enema (large-volume soap, oil) may all sometimes be necessary.

Faecal incontinence due to spinal or autonomic disease, often made worse by nocturnal sphincter atonia may be helped by codeine or morphine.

Sexual Function

Parasympathetic sacral nerve stimulation causes erection by vasodilatation, and sympathetic stimulation prevents erection by vasoconstriction. Ejaculation results from sympathetic stimulation of the vasa deferentia, seminal vesicles and prostate.

Many drugs interfere with libido, erection or ejaculation by both central and peripheral effects. Alcohol, cyproterone and oestrogens in males will reduce libido. Cocaine, yohimbine and amphetamine have a mythical reputation as aphrodisiacs, and cannabis may enhance sexual desire, although it causes a reduction in male serum testosterone levels. Levodopa will increase previously existent sexually deviant behaviour, but rarely alters libido.

Ejaculation may be delayed or prevented by neuroleptics, hypotensive drugs, including adrenergic neurone blockers and α-methyldopa, but not usually by beta-blockers and tricyclic antidepressants. Premature ejaculation may improve with clomipramine 10–15 mg nightly, or thioridazine 10–50 mg daily. Drug treatment of neurogenic impotence is unsatisfactory (but see p. 172). Androgens have no place, although bromocriptine will restore normal libido as well as fertility when infertility is due to hyperprolactinaemia.

Drugs and the Eye

The Pupil

Drug effects on the pupil can be helpful in assessing the adequacy of drugs given in neurological treatment. Many drugs with a cholinergic muscarinic blocking action (Table 10.3) cause cycloplegia and mydriasis. Anticholinesterases (neostigmine, physostigmine) cause miosis, which can indicate overtreatment in myasthenia.

Table 10.3. Some commonly used drugs which have a cholinergic muscarinic blocking action, causing mydriasis and loss of accommodation

Drug group	Examples
Antiparkinsonian	Benzhexol
	Benztropine
	Orphenadrine
Ulcer healing drugs	Hyoscine
	Dicyclomine
	Propantheline
Antihistamines	Mepyramine
	Mebhydrolin
	Chlorpheniramine
Major tranquillisers	Chlorpromazine
	Fluphenazine
	Promazine
	Prochlorperazine
	and others
Antidepressants	Amitriptyline
	Imipramine
	Trimipramine
	and others
Motion sickness drugs	Hyoscine
	Promethazine
	Dimenhydrinate

Drugs which block the synthesis or release of NA (including methyldopa and reserpine), or block ·NA receptors (phenoxybenzamine, phentolamine) cause miosis and ptosis (a pharmacological Horner's syndrome) by reducing sympathetic tone in the iris and upper lid. Ganglion-blockers, now rarely used, which block transmission at both sympathetic and parasympathetic ganglia, usually result in mydriasis and cycloplegia, as parasympathetic tone is normally dominant.

Toxic Effects of Drugs on the Eye

Intraocular

Disturbed Colour Vision (Chromatopsia)

Cardiac glycosides, some antimalarials (e.g. quinine, chloroquine), sulphona-mides, streptomycin, barbiturates and phenacetin can cause a yellowing of vision (xanthopsia) by action at an unknown (probably retinal) site.

Toxicity to the Lens and Conjunctiva

High-dosage steroid treatment can cause posterior subcapsular cataract originating as vacuolar change at the posterior pole. This was most commonly seen when high-dose steroids were the mainstay treatment after renal transplantation, with a total dose of 2–14 g prednisone in 3–12 months.

Phenothiazines (e.g. chlorpromazine) can leave photosensitive metabolite complexes in the lens, which are then activated by light so that an axial cataract develops. This rarely causes significant visual loss. Nitrogen mustard given by carotid perfusion can give rise to ipsilateral uveitis.

Glaucoma

In narrow-angle glaucoma, attacks of glaucoma can be precipitated by mydriatic drugs, such as antidepressants (e.g. amitriptyline, nortriptyline) and antiparkinsonian drugs with an anticholinergic action (e.g. benzhexol, benztropine). Steroids increase intraocular pressure by reducing aqueous outflow, so may aggravate both narrow-angle and open-angle glaucoma. Levodopa, at least in theory, may aggravate the severity of narrow-angle glaucoma.

Retinotoxicity

Quinine, chloroquine and ergots can rarely cause peripheral field constric-tion, whilst retinotoxicity from ethambutol, chloramphenicol, sulphona-mides, oral hypoglycaemics, penicillamine and tobacco results mainly in central field defects.

Chloroquine in low doses, like quinine, causes xanthopsia. Chloroquine disrupts vitamin A metabolism in the retina by inhibition of sulphydryl dehydrogenase, and accumulates selectively in the pigment epithelium. Loss of dark adaptation, disturbance of colour vision and central scotoma results. With prolonged use or high blood levels a retinopathy with macular degeneration and optic atrophy can often occur, with visual loss which may continue to progress on stopping the drug. Analogues of chloroquine (e.g. hydroxychloroquine, primaquine, mepacrine) can also cause a retinopathy.

Ethambutol in high dosage may deplete Cu and Zn from the retina. These metals act as prosthetic groups for retinol dehydrogenase in the pigment epithelium, and their loss may be associated with a toxic optic neuropathy and visual loss. This retinopathy is rare when ethambutol is limited to 16 mg kg^{-1} day^{-1} (unless the retina is otherwise compromised, as in diabetes). Visual loss following ethambutol treatment is usually partially or completely reversible, although it may progress for several months after stopping the drug. Like ethambutol, isoniazid can cause an optic neuropathy, although this is uncommon and confined to slow acetylators.

Indomethacin can cause a reversible retinopathy with impaired dark adaptation, macular pigmentation and optic disc pallor, probably through inhibition of lysosomal activity in the retina.

Steroids in high dosage may cause a patchy retinal oedema with scotoma. This is believed to be secondary to a steroid-induced hypertension, since it resolves when BP is lowered. Steroid treatment (particularly in children) can cause papilloedema.

Ethanol and methanol are oxidised by retinol dehydrogenase, forming acetaldehyde and formaldehyde, which are then oxidised to acetic and formic acid. Methanol is metabolised much more slowly than ethanol, but formaldehyde can cause permanent blindness. The treatment for methanol poisoning therefore includes giving ethanol (25 ml 50% p.o. 3-hourly), so as to saturate the enzyme with ethanol, and bicarbonate infusion to correct acidosis. Haemodialysis may be needed.

Tobacco–alcohol amblyopia has been associated with cyanide toxicity due to vitamin B_{12} deficiency. Cobalamines have a high affinity for cyanides, which occur in high amounts in some tobaccos. This affinity may result in deficiency of active vitamin B_{12}, as well as failure of detoxification of cyanide. However, treatment of tobacco amblyopia with hydroxocobalamine does not usually restore vision.

In high doses, piperidine-substituted phenothiazines (e.g. thioridazine, 800–1000 mg daily) can cause pigmentary retinal stippling and plaques, and in addition retinal artery narrowing, resulting in central visual loss. These changes are usually reversible on stopping treatment.

Retrobulbar Neuritis

Chloramphenicol can rarely cause retrobulbar as well as peripheral neuritis, but it is usually reversible if treatment is stopped promptly when it occurs.

Oculomotor Toxic Effects

Acute Dystonia

Phenothiazines and substituted benzamides cause acute dystonic reactions, which may include oculogyric crises, in about 5% of people. Oculogyric crises (forced involuntary upward deviation of the eyes, sometimes with partial eye closure), occur particularly in children. Drugs such as perphenazine, prochlorperazine and metoclopramide may be responsible during initial dosage (commonly after the first 1–2 doses). Acute dystonia may last from a few hours to several days, with focal or general dystonia as well as oculogyric crises. Diazepam 2–10 mg i.v. (adult dose) or benztropine mesylate 1–2 mg i.m. or i.v. will rapidly abolish such drug-induced acute dystonic reactions.

Oculovestibular Effects

Benzodiazepines, barbiturates, other hypnotics and alchohol will all cause weakening of convergence and a breakdown of pursuit movements, with gaze-evoked nystagmus. Phenytoin in mildly toxic doses (20–40 mg/l) causes nystagmus on lateral gaze. At higher levels vertical nystagmus on upward gaze, second-degree nystagmus and gaze palsy (40–60 mg/l), and finally external ophthalmoplegia (over 60 mg/l) progressively occur.

Ocular Motor Neuropathies

Nitrofurantoin can cause polyneuritis including cranial nerve palsies with pareses of extraocular muscles. This is usually associated with excessive blood levels, so nitrofurantoin is avoided if renal function is impaired.

Toxic Neuromuscular Blockade of Intraocular Muscles

Tricyclic antidepressants with anticholinergic effects, and anticholinergic drugs used in the treatment of parkinsonism, urge incontinence and in the prevention of gastrointestinal side effects of anticholinesterases, may cause paresis of accommodation and mydriasis. This results in complaints of blurred vision and occasionally of being dazzled.

Toxic Neuromuscular Blockade of Extraocular Muscles

Excess dosage of neostigmine or pyridostigmine in myasthenia can cause a depolarising blockade of the neuromuscular junction of extraocular muscles, resulting in an increase, rather than decrease, in severity of fatiguable diplopia. In practice, it is usually impossible to determine the occurrence of this depolarising blockade from ocular observations alone. Attention must be concentrated on bulbar and respiratory function, and its response to edrophonium.

Raised Intracranial Pressure

Steroid or surgical treatment of raised intracranial pressure results in commencement of resolution of papilloedema with a delay on average of about 1–3 days. With acute papilloedema, complete resolution of disc changes may occur within 1 week.

Rapid withdrawal of steroids given for other reasons (e.g. temporal arteritis), and particularly in children can result in intracranial hypertension and papilloedema. If this occurs, steroids should be restarted, followed by a slower withdrawal.

In infants, nalidixic acid and tetracycline can occasionally cause intracranial hypertension and papilloedema, as can either excess or deficiency of vitamin A in both children and adults. Very rarely, the contraceptive pill has been associated with intracranial hypertension and papilloedema, particularly in obese women. This rare occurrence may not be related to contraceptive progesterone intake at all, but be due to the coincidence of benign intracranial hypertension.

Extraocular

Ocular Myasthenia

The extraocular muscles are often affected early and severely in myasthenia gravis, causing diplopia and ptosis. One or more individual muscles may be affected. Treatment with anticholinesterase drugs (neostigmine, pyridostigmine) is needed if ocular symptoms are frequent, continuous or troublesome, or if there are symptoms of muscle fatigue elsewhere (myasthenia gravis). If myasthenia gravis is severe, immunosuppressants with or without thymectomy are often added. Even when control of myasthenia is otherwise good, with no generalised weakness, it is rare to achieve complete freedom from diplopia using anticholinesterases alone.

Treatment with many drugs which possess neuromuscular blocking activity or act on skeletal muscle may increase the severity of ocular myasthenia: these include aminoglycosides, propranolol and guanine.

Further Reading

Bannister RW (ed) (1983) Autonomic failure: a textbook of clinical disorders of the autonomic nervous system. Oxford University Press, Oxford
Brindley GS, Polkey CE, Rushton DN, Cardozo L (1986) Sacral anterior root stimulators: report of the first 50 cases. J Neurol Neurosurg Psychiatry

11 Drugs in Neuroendocrinology

Corticosteroids and ACTH

Corticosteroids reduce antibody formation, and have an anti-inflammatory effect. The main use of these drugs in neurology is to suppress disease processes. Although corticosteroids are widely used in many different neurological disorders, their value is sometimes uncertain. The main indications are set out in Table 11.1.

Steroids in Multiple Sclerosis

Long-term trials of corticosteroids and also other immunosuppressive drugs in multiple sclerosis have been mainly done because of common features between experimental allergic encephalomyelitis and multiple sclerosis. However, the lesions of allergic encephalomyelitis differ pathologically from those of multiple sclerosis, and the two conditions have a different course, the former resulting in either recovery or death. ACTH, prednisolone, antilymphocytic globulin and azathioprine have all been investigated. The overall results have been very disappointing, with no unequivocal evidence of worthwhile improvement, although a few well-controlled studies have suggested that the number of relapses in early multiple sclerosis can be reduced by corticosteroids. However, there is no real evidence of any reduction of overall disease progression, and occasionally steroids have to be stopped because of intercurrent infection or gastric irritation.

The production of IgG in the central nervous system appears to be related to the production of lesions in multiple sclerosis, and occurs in over 90% of patients with clinically definite multiple sclerosis. ACTH gel, or the combination of ACTH with prednisolone, will suppress IgG formation. (Dexamethasone is possibly less effective than ACTH–prednisolone combinations in this respect.) A short course of ACTH produces rapid and long-lasting suppression of IgG synthesis. However, in multiple sclerosis, short- or long-term ACTH treatment does not produce any definite alteration in

Table 11.1. Probable therapeutic value of glucocorticosteroids in various neurological disorders (Wiles 1982)

Therapeutic value	Disorder
Definite	Perifocal oedema/raised intracranial pressure secondary to intrinsic subacute/chronic mass lesion, for example tumour (major temporary benefit)
	Compression of neural structures by a subacute/chronic extrinsic lesion (minor temporary benefit)
	Perioperative use for neurosurgery
	Giant cell arteritis (definitive treatment)
	Myasthenia gravis (definitive treatment sometimes)
	Polymyositis (definitive treatment)
	Others (for example hypsarrhythmia)
Uncertain	Traumatic brain/spinal cord injury of acute type
	Meningitis/encephalitis, due to viral and bacterial (including tuberculosis) causes
	Benign intracranial hypertension
	Stroke
	Optic neuritis and multiple sclerosis
	Bell's palsy
	Acute inflammatory and chronic relapsing polyneuropathy
	Myasthenic syndrome
	Neurological complications of systemic disease, for example collagen vascular disease, sarcoidosis
None	Diffuse brain swelling due to metabolic insult, for example hypoxia and water intoxication
	Cerebral malaria

chronic or progressive disability, and cerebrospinal fluid oligoclonal bands are not eradicated (Tourtellotte et al. 1980).

Dowling et al. (1980) gave very high doses of intravenous and then oral steroids (methylprednisolone 125–300 mg i.v. 6-hourly for 2–4 days followed by oral therapy—a very expensive regime) to patients with multiple sclerosis, and claimed substantial improvement within 3–4 days. However, this trial was uncontrolled.

Half of all patients with an acute demyelinating optic neuritis develop subsequent multiple sclerosis. Rawson et al. (1966, 1969) showed that short courses of ACTH reduced ocular pain and resulted in earlier return of vision over 1 month, although there is no evidence that the routine use of ACTH or prednisolone in unilateral optic neuritis will alter the final outcome. In practice, most patients with acute retrobulbar neuritis are treated with short courses of ACTH.

Neither low- nor high-dose long-term glucocorticoid or ACTH therapy in multiple sclerosis is thought to prevent relapse. In the early 1960s, Miller et al. (1961, 1967) found no benefit from the extended use of either ACTH or glucocorticoids in multiple sclerosis.

As with steroids, most studies of transfer factor in multiple sclerosis have given negative results. Basten et al. (1980) gave mildly and severely affected victims of multiple sclerosis transfer factor obtained from the leucocytes of relatives, with about 20 injections over 2 years. Overall, transfer factor did not cause worthwhile improvement or clearly affect immune function. In mildly affected subjects, slightly less overall deterioration was found in patients given transfer factor as compared with placebo, but in those who were severely affected there was no improvement in illness or reduction in relapse rate. A placebo effect may be expected in up to one-third of all subjects with multiple sclerosis subjected to any major procedure.

A number of other orthodox as well as bizarre procedures have been investigated in patients with multiple sclerosis in an attempt to reduce disease progression. These include acupuncture, snake venom, hyperbaric oxygen and dorsal column stimulation. All of these procedures carry a definite hazard or produce discomfort or infection, and none can be recommended (Rosen and Barsoum 1979).

The use of hyperbaric oxygen in multiple sclerosis may stem from the occasional improvement in conscious level with this treatment seen in patients with severe head injury, raised intracranial pressure and anoxic brain damage (Suloff and Ragatz 1982). Here, hyperbaric oxygenation reduces cerebral cortical blood flow, without preventing elevation of cerebral oxygen tension, and appears to be helpful in the treatment of cerebral oedema. Presumably any effect is due to increasing the viability of damaged tissue. No definite value of hyperbaric oxygen in the treatment of multiple sclerosis has at present been demonstrated.

Steroids in Cerebral Oedema and Severe Head Injury

Steroids are of major although temporary benefit in patients with intrinsic malignant tumours causing focal neurological signs, and symptoms of raised intracranial pressure. The response is often dramatic when these features are due to peritumoral oedema, although there is probably no benefit to the primary lesion. Improvement may be gained for several months in lesions with extensive oedema. The action of natural and synthetic glucocorticoids in cerebral oedema with cerebral tumours may be due to restoration of normal capillary endothelial permeability. Dexamethasone, 2–4 mg 8-hourly p.o., which lacks mineralocorticoid activity, will reduce cerebral oedema within 2–4 h of starting treatment.

The use of steroids to reduce cerebral oedema following stroke and in head injury, or in benign lesions such as meningiomas which produce their effects mainly by direct pressure, is much more controversial. The effect of steroids in head injury is different in different patient groups, but in subjects with depressed skull fractures, intracerebral haematomas or cerebral contusion, any action is minor, and the immediate as well as the ultimate outcome is not greatly altered. Saul et al. (1981) gave patients with severe head injuries very high steroid dosages (dexamethasone 1 mg kg^{-1} day^{-1}) for an initial

3-day period, continuing for a further week if the overall condition improved, but withdrawing treatment if there was no obvious benefit. This approach did not affect overall mortality, although a few subjects may have gained some immediate benefit. However, when intracranial pressure is raised following head injury, the use of controlled ventilation and osmotic agents such as mannitol is probably of more value than glucocorticoids.

In patients with benign intracranial hypertension as a result of increased resistance to the flow of CSF from the subarachnoid space into the dural villi, and in whom weight reduction and lumbar puncture do not relieve symptoms, the use of glucocorticoids usually results in rapid symptomatic resolution.

Following brain infarction, brain swelling occurs and is maximal from 36 h to 4 days after the acute event. Oedema results from both cellular metabolic impairment in the damaged area (cytotoxic oedema) and expansion of the extracellular space owing to leakage of colloid ("vasogenic" oedema). There is loss of local vascular autoregulation. It is still not clear whether glucocorticoids are of value in ischaemic infarction. If there is progressive focal brain swelling following infarction, and progressive clinical deterioration occurs, dexamethasone may be justified, but there is no rationale for giving steroids to all patients with stroke.

Bell's Palsy

Spontaneous and complete recovery occurs in 60% of all cases of Bell's palsy seen within the first 6 days of illness, and these patients do not need any treatment. However, it is difficult if not impossible to identify subjects who will develop denervation, serious contractures, or aberrant reinnervation. These features may be most common in the elderly, or those with complete paralysis when first seen. If this group could be clearly identified, some form of treatment would be highly desirable. Despite several trials, it has not been clearly shown that glucocorticoids or ACTH will prevent these complications. Many clinicians give a short course of either ACTH or prednisolone to cases of Bell's palsy presenting within the first 10 days, unless there are contraindications, in the hope that this may improve the final outcome in the small proportion of cases who would not otherwise completely recover.

Acute Inflammatory and Chronic Relapsing Polyneuropathy

Most cases of acute inflammatory polyneuropathy recover spontaneously and are left with little or no residual disability, and there is no clear evidence that either prednisolone in high dosage, or ACTH given in the initial stage of illness, has a major effect on the acute disease. Indeed, the use of glucocorticoids may possibly impair spontaneous recovery, although the data, at least in mild cases, is conflicting.

A minority of patients initially diagnosed as having acute inflammatory polyneuropathy do not recover, or relapse after initial recovery. It is not clear whether acute and chronic idiopathic polyneuropathies are different diseases, or due to differences in the host immune response. In patients with the chronic form of illness, glucocorticoids are often highly effective, although dose reduction or drug withdrawal may be followed by relapse (see pp. 160, 161).

In contrast to steroids, plasmapheresis appears to be of definite value in the management of acute inflammatory polyneuropathy, although the procedure is not entirely without risk. Early plasmapheresis may offer the best chance for reducing morbidity.

Other Uses of Steroids in Neurology

Hypophysectomy

Hydrocortisone is needed (but not fludrocortisone, since aldosterone production is dependent on the renin–angiotensin system rather than on ACTH). Thyroid, sex hormones and growth hormone should also be given as indicated.

Immune Suppression

In diseases such as polyarteritis nodosa, polymyositis or myasthenia gravis, or in inflammatory disorders (e.g. meningitis) selectivity of glucocorticoid rather than mineralocorticoid effect is needed (see Table 11.4). High-dosage prednisolone, e.g. 20 mg 8-hourly, is usually given to start treatment, although in myasthenia, steroid treatment should commence with an alternate-day, low-dosage regime, to avoid the possible provocation of a crisis (see p. 157).

Postural Hypotension

The aldosterone-like effect of fludrocortisone, with salt and water retention and expansion of extracellular fluid volume, many be of value here, although the head up/feet down sleep posture, catecholamine infusion and sympathomimetic drugs are usually more effective (but see p. 169).

Hypsarrhythmia

Both ACTH and corticosteroids are occasionally successful. The mechanism is not known.

Dexamethasone Suppression Test

Glucocorticoids suppress the hypothalamic–pituitary–adrenal axis, and the effect is greatest and most prolonged at night. In normal subjects, dexamethasone 1 mg will suppress ACTH secretion for 24 h. ACTH suppression by dexamethasone does not occur in Cushing's disease.

Cushing's Disease and Syndrome

Medical treatment may be attempted if the patient is too ill for surgery or refuses radiation. Metyrapone, 0.75–4 g daily, blocks 11-β-hydroxylation. Aminoglutethimide, 250 mg 8-hourly, inhibits the production of pregnenolone from cholesterol and blocks all steroid synthesis. Mitotane (o,p-DDT) has a direct toxic effect on adrenal tumours, and also on pulmonary metastases. Cyproheptadine has a central effect, and reduces ACTH secretion. Tranquillisers, morphine and antidepressants cause a minor reduction in ACTH release.

Dexamethasone Suppression Test in Endogenous Depression

In endogenous depression, both the timing and the control of cortisol release are abnormal in up to 70% of all subjects. The usual findings are an overall increase in mean 24-h urinary free cortisol concentration, and an increase in the degree of diurnal variation of plasma cortisol levels. Peak plasma cortisol levels may occur 3–4 h earlier than usual, i.e. at 3.00 a.m. instead of 7.00 a.m., perhaps due to the marked sleep disruption of these subjects. Associated with this, dexamethasone suppression of cortisol release is sometimes impaired in subjects with endogenous depression. Whatever the mechanism, variation in plasma cortisol level and impaired dexamethasone suppression of cortisol release return to normal with treatment and recovery of endogenous depression.

Addison's Disease or Following Adrenalectomy

Cortisone acetate has been replaced by the active metabolite hydrocortisone, 20–30 mg p.o. daily, divided into larger morning and smaller evening dosage to mimic natural cortisone production. Alternatively, prednisone or prednisolone may be used. These drugs have appreciable mineralocorticoid activity, but need to be reinforced with fludrocortisone 50–200 μg daily.

Anabolic Steroids

The protein-building property of anabolic steroids led to the hope that they may be of value in muscle-wasting diseases and muscle dystrophy. This hope has not been realised. The anabolic steroid nandrolone may be of value in promoting protein synthesis after major surgery, and in the control of osteoporosis, but is not of proven value in any primary neuromuscular disorder. Some other anabolic steroids (e.g. ethyloestrenol) may cause cholestatic jaundice or hepatic tumours in long-term use, and these drugs are not recommended in any neurological disorder.

Pharmacology of Corticosteroids and ACTH (Table 11.2)

Corticosteroids

The main adrenal cortex steroids are hydrocortisone (cortisol), corticosterone, aldosterone and dehydroepiandrosterone. These have widespread actions on carbohydrate and protein metabolism, sodium balance and extracellular fluid volume, and sexual function. Hormone synthesis from the precursor cholesterol is continuous, with little adrenal storage. However, drugs that reduce plasma cholesterol levels do not impair steroid synthesis. The normal release of adrenal steroids is pulsatile over 24 h, both sleeping and waking, and is under pituitary control via release of ACTH (corticotropin).

ACTH

ACTH, with 39 amino acid residues, is structurally similar to melanocyte-stimulating hormone (MSH), and is released from the anterior pituitary in response to hypothalamic corticotropin-releasing hormones. ACTH determines cortisol, but not aldosterone production.

Tetracosactrin is a synthetic ACTH analogue, containing the first 24 amino acids of ACTH, which are similar in all species. Both drugs are inactive by mouth. Injection in water produces only a brief effect, 15–30 min. Depot preparations, e.g. ACTH 40–100 units, or tetracosactrin 0.5–1 mg, given daily, cause a more sustained elevation of cortisol levels.

In the pituitary, ACTH, lipotropin, opioid peptides and the melanotropins, come from a common precursor. The role of these different compounds, including α- and γ-MSH, the endorphins and related peptides, is not established in humans, and none of these compounds or their analogues has a definite established place or superiority to corticosteroids in the treatment of any neurological or psychiatric disorder.

Endorphins

In 1973 it was found that radioactive opiates bind to tropine receptors in membranes, and have a regional distribution in pain pathways. Subsequently two pentapeptides called enkephalins, with opiate activity, were isolated from brain and pituitary. The amino acid sequence of one of these, Met-enkephalin,

Table 11.2. Comparison of effects of ACTH and corticosteroids[a]

ACTH	Corticosteroids
Lacks selective glucocorticoid effect	Selective glucocorticoid activity
Adrenal cortex stimulation unpredictable and limited to four times normal output	Effects dose-related with different drugs. Potent and rapid-acting compounds available
Stimulates androgen release	May have no androgenic effect
Minor increase in aldosterone	May have little or no mineralocorticoid activity
Causes adrenal hypertrophy	Cause adrenal atrophy

[a] The alleged differences between ACTH and corticosteroids in short-term neurological treatment may be imaginary, as comparable doses producing similar urinary 17-oxogenic steroid excretion have not been compared.

is identical to the 61–65 residue of betalipotropin. Other portions of betalipotropin were then shown to have similar effects, and these polypeptides are called endorphins, an abbreviation for endogenous morphine.

Pituitary hormonal effects of these opiate peptides are similar to those of morphine, with growth hormone, prolactin and ADH release, and inhibition of luteinising hormone. The behavioural and motor, as well as endocrine actions of opioid peptides, have been widely investigated, although at present no role in the treatment of any neurological or psychiatric disorder has been established.

Clinical Management of Corticosteroid Treatment in Neurology

Acute steroid treatment with systemic hydrocortisone hemisuccinate 100–500 mg i.v. can be life-saving in severe shock, particularly with Gram-negative septicaemia in meningococcal meningitis (see p. 102).

Short (7–14 day) corticosteroid courses are usually without serious adverse effect, but may alter subcutaneous fat distribution and cause the moon face of Cushing's syndrome and, rarely, may produce major changes in mood and personality, or precipitate hypokalaemia and digitalis toxicity.

Long-term corticosteroid treatment (months or years) often produces serious side effects (Table 11.3), and is only indicated to save or prolong life, to relieve severe disability in myasthenia or polymyositis, or prevent serious complications such as ciliary artery thrombosis leading to blindness in temporal arteritis. Maintenance dosage should be kept as low as possible, i.e. prednisolone 2.5–10 mg daily or on alternate days. On stopping the drug, corticosteroids should be withdrawn gradually over 1–8 weeks, depending on the length of previous therapy.

The risks of steroids (Table 11.3) are greater in children than in adults, and growth may be stunted. Risks can be minimised by giving prednisolone on alternate days. Short courses of ACTH are usually without serious risk, but very occasionally ACTH and tetracosactrin, given in depot preparations, produce allergic reactions.

Table 11.3. Disadvantages of steroids

System	Disadvantage
Immunological	Diminished immunoglobulin production, spread or masking of infection
Nervous system	Euphoria, depression, paranoia and other psychiatric changes. These are usually dose-related, and most frequent in patients with a history of previous mental disorder
Skeletal	Backache, osteoporosis, renal calculi, failure of growth in children
Visual	Change in focus, posterior capsular cataract
Alimentary	Dyspepsia, peptic ulceration and haemorrhage
Cardiovascular	Hypertension, atherosclerosis
Haematological	Polycythaemia, florid complexion
Water and salt metabolism	Sodium retention, potassium loss, muscle weakness, particularly with fluorinated steroids, triamcinolone, betamethasone and dexamethasone
General metabolism	Cushing's syndrome, weight gain, redistribution of body fat, moon face, myopathy

A number of different corticosteroid preparations are available, with different ratios of anti-inflammatory to mineralocorticoid activity (Table 11.4). The choice of preparation depends on clinical indication.

Table 11.4. Corticosteroid equivalents

Drug	Equivalent dose (mg)	Ratio anti-inflammatory: mineralocorticoid activity
Betamethasone	1	25:0[d]
Dexamethasone[a]	1	25:0[d]
Methylprednisolone	5	5:0.5
Prednisone[b]	5	4:0.8
Prednisolone[c]	7	4:0.8
Hydrocortisone	25	1:1
Cortisone acetate	33	0.8:1
Fludrocortisone	2	1:500

[a] Can cause negative calcium balance
[b] More expensive, and great individual variation in conversion to its active derivative, prednisolone
[c] Enteric-coated preparations available with identical bioavailability, but little evidence of any difference in gastric irritation
[d] Minimal mineralocorticoid activity

Pharmacokinetics of Corticosteroids (Table 11.5)

Steroids are rapidly absorbed when given p.o., with peak plasma levels at 1–3 h. The absorption of cortisone acetate given intramuscularly is slower than when given by mouth, and absorption is sometimes erratic. The bioavailability of prednisolone is greater than that of prednisone.

Table 11.5. Pharmacokinetics of steroids

Drug	Absorption		Distribution		Elimination	
	Fraction (%)	t_{max} (h)	V_d (l/kg)	Binding (%)	$t_{1/2}$ (h)	Unchanged (%)
Cortisone	Good	Rapid p.o., slower i.m.	Wide	100	0.5	Conjugated
Hydrocortisone	Good	Rapid	Wide	90	1–2	1
Fludrocortisone	Good	1.5–2	Wide	70–80		Hydrolysed
Prednisone	Good	1	Wide	50	3	Converted to prednisolone
Prednisolone	Good	1	Wide	50	3	10–30 (mostly conjugated)
Dexamethasone	Good	1	Wide	77	2–5	65
Betamethasone	Good	1	Wide	65	2–5	65

Mean plasma cortisol levels vary over 24 h, high at 8.00 a.m. (6–25 μg per 100 ml) and low at midnight (less than 8 μg per 100 ml). When used for replacement therapy, hydrocortisone should be given in a larger morning than evening dose, to replicate this natural pattern. Otherwise, when corticosteroids are used in immunosuppression or for treatment of cerebral oedema, 8-hourly equal doses should be given; once daily in maintenance therapy.

Cortisol is 95% plasma-bound. With high cortisol levels, the percentage of free cortisol may rise. Adverse effects are correlated with the amount of free drug, and in patients with low plasma albumin, dosage should be reduced. In pregnancy, the protein binding of cortisol increases.

The plasma half-life of cortisol is 100–150 min, although the biological effects last 8–12 h. The plasma half-life is increased in cirrhosis and myxoedema, and reduced in thyrotoxicosis. With a single intramuscular dose of hydrocortisone 200 mg, a clinical effect is usually apparent after 1 h, although a single dose may not have any useful neurological effect for 8 h after administration.

Plasma cortisol level determination is not of value in the management of neurological disease, except to assess the results of replacement therapy or the action of suppressive drugs in Cushing's syndrome. Plasma steroid levels do not correlate with the long-term biological effect, although they may relate to acute toxic actions. The determination of urinary 17-ketogenic or 17-oxogenic steroid levels (depending on laboratory method) is of more value.

Steroid Interactions

Steroids antagonise the antidiabetic action of insulin and oral hypoglycaemic drugs. The mineralocorticoid effect of corticosteroids will increase the potassium-losing effects of diuretics such as frusemide. Antiepileptic drugs which increase the activity of hepatic microsomal enzyme systems can increase the metabolism of steroids and reduce the clinical effect. Salicylates and phenylbutazone compete with steroids for plasma protein-binding sites, and will increase the amount of free steroids.

Steroid Withdrawal

Sudden steroid withdrawal may lead to acute adrenal deficiency and, for 1–2 years after steroid withdrawal, stress, operation or infection may precipitate a crisis and require administration of steroids, electrolytes, glucose and water. Acute steroid withdrawal may rarely cause raised intracranial pressure and papilloedema.

Treatment of Pituitary Tumours

Prolactin-Secreting Adenomas

Small pituitary adenomas are found in over 9% of autopsies, although most of these are probably asymptomatic in life. The commonest functional pituitary tumour is a prolactin-secreting adenoma. Most of these are small, and do not cause pressure symptoms, although they are a common and important cause of infertility, accounting for between 20% and 30% of all cases. Hyperprolactinaemia results in infertility, with blockade of the action of gonadotropins on the gonads.

The detection of a small prolactin-producing adenoma as the cause of hyperprolactinaemia and infertility can be difficult, and requires the demonstration of loss of both the normal circadian rhythm of prolactin production, and loss of the normal response to thyrotropin-releasing hormone and metoclopramide, as well as detailed skull tomography. Large adenomas cause obvious pituitary fossa defects and very high prolactin levels, as well as producing optic nerve compression.

Until recently, the first line of approach to these tumours was surgery or radiotherapy. Transsphenoidal microdissection of small adenomas is often curative, and restores normal fertility with no notable complications. However, surgery (or radiotherapy) may interfere with other pituitary-dependent hormones, prolactin levels do not always return to normal, and gland size may not diminish for 6 months after irradiation.

It has recently been shown that dopamine agonist ergot derivatives (e.g. bromocriptine 10–60 mg daily, pergolide 2–6 mg or lisuride 1–4 mg) cause immediate and sustained prolactin suppression, often with rapid restoration of fertility, and without interference with gonadotropins. In addition, there may be a reduction in tumour size, and resolution of visual field defects. However, some pituitary adenomas continue to enlarge, particularly during pregnancy, despite the use of ergot alkaloids, and visual field analysis in pituitary adenomas must continue despite this treatment. On balance, the present evidence suggests that the initial treatment of pituitary prolactinomas which do not compromise vision should be medical, not surgical.

Drugs such as bromocriptine restore fertility when this is lost owing to hyperprolactinaemia, but not when infertility is the result of other causes. Bromocriptine lowers prolactin levels and restores fertility, with return of normal menstruation and ovulation in women, and libido and potency in men, in most cases within 4–12 weeks of starting treatment. Response is occasionally delayed for up to 6 months.

Pituitary Tumours in Pregnancy

The management of pituitary tumours in pregnancy is difficult. In infertile women with microprolactinomas and hyperprolactinaemia treated with bromocriptine, restoration of fertility and subsequent pregnancy are often rapid. The normal pituitary almost doubles in size during pregnancy, and the potential for a pituitary tumour to compromise vision during pregnancy is very considerable. Because of this, irradiation of big tumours, despite absence of compressive symptoms, is sometimes advised before commencing bromocriptine treatment in infertile women of child-bearing age with prolactinomas. Even if this policy is adopted, repeated visual charting for evidence of nerve or chiasmal compression is necessary throughout pregnancy.

Although hyperprolactinaemia is often due to a pituitary adenoma, nontumorous causes of pathological hyperprolactinaemia are common, resulting in galactorrhoea and infertility. Galactorrhoea may result from dopamine receptor antagonist drugs (e.g. chlorpromazine), dopamine-depleting drugs (e.g. reserpine), hypothalamic–pituitary disease, myxoedema or chronic renal disease. In all these conditions, bromocriptine 5–20 mg daily, given 8-hourly, restores prolactin levels to normal, and stops milk production, often within 1 week. Higher doses of bromocriptine, up to 50 mg daily, are sometimes necessary if galactorrhoea results from intense dopamine receptor blockade due to neuroleptic drugs, or if initial prolactin levels are very high with a large prolactin-secreting adenoma.

The natural history of pituitary adenomas is uncertain, and spontaneous remission without treatment may sometimes occur. Although bromocriptine will suppress symptomatology for many years, with both prolactin- and growth hormone-secreting tumours, symptoms usually recur if the drug is stopped, and treatment may not be curative.

Acromegaly

The treatment of acromegaly with ergot derivatives is not as successful as the treatment of prolactin-secreting adenomas. Bromocriptine 5–20 mg 8-hourly causes a sustained dose-related decrease in plasma growth hormone levels in most acromegalic subjects but, unlike prolactin, growth hormone levels rarely fall to normal values despite high doses of bromocriptine, and complete clinical remission occurs in only a minority of subjects, although most acromegalics show some degree of response. Headache, excessive sweating, sexual performance, soft tissue swelling, are all improved. The degree of clinical improvement in these subjects is often greater than would be expected from the fall in plasma growth hormone levels. Between 20% and 30% of acromegalics show an inadequate response, occasionally with drug intolerance or inadequate treatment period. Others who fail to improve may lack receptors for dopamine agonist drugs on growth hormone-secreting cells.

As with prolactinomas, ergot derivatives will reduce the size of growth hormone-producing pituitary adenomas, although the response here is less consistent than in the case of prolactin-secreting tumours, and surgery should still be considered if there is any suggestion of optic nerve compression or no obvious clinical improvement on the drug. Medical treatment occasionally results in haemorrhage or infarction into the tumour, with pituitary apoplexy. Prolonged suppression of growth hormone secretion in acromegaly has been obtained using a somatostatin analogue, although somatostatin itself, which has a very short half-life, is ineffective clinically.

Mode of Action of Ergot Derivatives in Hyperprolactinaemia and Acromegaly

Under normal conditions, dopamine is released by the hypothalamus, and acts as a physiologically active prolactin inhibitory factor. Exogenous levodopa, and dopamine agonist drugs, are equally effective, although the action of the ergot derivatives is usually more prolonged than that of levodopa.

Levodopa, bromocriptine and other ergot derivatives cause a brief rise in plasma growth hormone levels in normal subjects, probably due to a hypothalamic action, but a sustained fall in plasma growth hormone levels in patients with acromegaly, probably owing to a direct inhibitory effect on the pituitary. There is little effect on other pituitary hormones, although bromocriptine occasionally inhibits ACTH production in Cushing's disease and Nelson's syndrome, and also inhibits MSH release. In normal subjects, neuroleptic drugs have opposite hormonal effects to those of dopamine agonists, and growth hormone release is inhibited by phenothiazines, butyrophenones, reserpine, tetrabenazine, α-methyldopa and p-amino-methyltyrosine.

The pituitary hormonal effects of dopamine-like drugs are of little or no practical importance in elderly patients with Parkinson's disease, and it is unlikely that growth failure in children on neuroleptic medication is the result of growth hormone deficiency.

Growth Failure

Failure to grow may result from end-organ resistance to growth hormone (African Pygmy); production of growth hormone with normal immunological but no biological activity; or failure of production of the growth hormone factors (somatomedins). Growth hormone underproduction may be sporadic, familial, due to hypopituitarism, or the result of emotional deprivation and neglect in children. Foetal growth hormone is not necessary for foetal growth.

Treatment of growth hormone deficiency in children with active soma-tomedins may replace the use of growth hormone. At present, treatment should be confined to children with open epiphyses. Growth hormone prepared by recombinant technology will be available shortly. The use of growth hormone prepared from human post-mortem material has been associated with the subsequent development of Jakob–Creutzfeldt disease, and these preparations should not be used.

Antidiuretic Hormone

Antidiuretic hormone (ADH, vasopressin) is used to treat diabetes insipidus of hypothalamic–pituitary origin. It is not of value in nephrogenic diabetes insipidus, where ADH levels are normal but the renal tubular response is impaired. ADH is usually given as 8-lysine vasopressin (lypressin) or the longer-acting ADH analogue desmopressin, which does not have any vasoconstrictor effect. When diabetes insipidus follows pituitary surgery or head injury, ADH, if required, is usually necessary only in small doses over a limited period. As an alternative to ADH, in mild cases of diabetes insipidus of central origin, chlorpropamide will reduce polyuria, although it carries a risk of hypoglycaemia.

Naturally occurring ADH is arginine vasopressin in most mammalian species. It is nonapeptide released from nerve endings of paraventricular neurones under the control of noradrenaline and acetylcholine. ADH acts on the kidney to reduce water loss. The pressor actions of ADH require 100 times larger doses than those causing maximal antidiuresis, but in high doses ADH constricts the coronary blood vessels, and may cause angina.

ADH is prepared by synthesis or from the posterior pituitary gland of domestic animals, separated from oxytocin. ADH is rapidly inactivated by peptidases, and removed by the kidney, and longer-acting preparations are available. Lypressin is 8-lysine vasopressin (5–20 units intranasally 3–7 times a day). Desmopressin (DDAVP) has a prolonged half-life. DDAVP 10–20 μg (adult dose) absorbed through the nasal mucous membrane will produce antidiuresis for 12 h, 0.5–2 μg given i.m. will produce antidiuresis for 24 h. The i.m. route is used mainly for the initial diagnosis of diabetes insipidus, and also postoperatively. The dose of DDAVP should be determined by the individual response, and diuresis should not be completely suppressed, in order to avoid water intoxication.

In addition to their antidiuretic actions, these compounds all have nonrenal effects, and cause nasal congestion, ulceration, hypertension, asthma, hypersensitivity, a desire to defecate, coronary vasospasm and angina. They may also have minor effects on learning behaviour and memory consolidation, although these are not clinically important, and no defect in memory has been shown in subjects who lack ADH.

Hyperosmolarity, stress, an upright posture and hypotension, increase ADH release under normal circumstances. Excess ADH secretion in relation to plasma osmolarity (inappropriate ADH secretion syndrome—resulting in water retention, hyponatraemia and very high plasma ADH levels) may result from drugs which stimulate ADH secretion (e.g. vincristine, cyclophosphamide, clofibrate, chlorpropamide, tricyclic antidepressants, carbamazepine and morphine) or result from ectopic hormone production by tumours, head injury and chest disease. Hypo-osmolarity, hypertension, a recumbent posture, alcohol, phenytoin and anticholinergic drugs cause a decrease in ADH production.

Chlorpropamide and tolbutamide, but not other sulphonylureas, enhance the action of ADH on the kidney, and may stimulate ADH release. They are not effective when there is a complete absence of the hormone, and are useful only in mild cases of hypothalamic diabetes insipidus. Chlorpropamide requires about 3 days to produce its effect, and is potentially dangerous, particularly in patients with hypopituitarism, due to prolonged hypoglycaemia. These drugs have a limited role in the short-term treatment of diabetes insipidus following hypophysectomy, but dosage should be restricted to chlorpropamide 350 mg daily (adults) or 200 mg (children).

Thiazide diuretics have a paradoxical antidiuretic effect, and are clinically useful in ADH nonresponsive nephrogenic diabetes insipidus, especially if sodium intake is restricted, but not in diabetes insipidus of central origin. Oral potassium supplements should be given.

Lithium inhibits the action of ADH, and will produce polyuria and polydipsia. Weight gain with lithium is usually due to fluid retention.

Demeclocycline 600–1000 mg daily p.o., a tetracycline broad-spectrum antibiotic, is an ADH antagonist which blocks the effect of ADH on the renal tubule. Demeclocycline can produce polyuria and polydipsia, and will reverse the hyponatraemia of inappropriate ADH secretion.

Sex Hormones

Anti-androgens

Cyproterone

This anti-androgen blocks testosterone synthesis. Cyproterone acetate 50–100 mg 12-hourly will suppress sexual activity in men for 10–14 days. Only 10%–50% of an oral dose is absorbed, and metabolism is rapid, although the drug may suppress spermatogenesis for 6 months after withdrawal. Some 10% of subjects develop gynaecomastia, and daytime drowsiness is common, so patients on cyproterone should be warned not to drive. The drug is of value combined with levodopa or bromocriptine when these produce sexually deviant behaviour.

Diabetes Mellitus

Approximately 5% of the United Kingdom population have symptoms of diabetes mellitus, with a raised random blood glucose level, or an abnormal glucose tolerance test following glucose 75 g by mouth. Diabetes is associated with frequent neurological complications, including neuropathy, stroke and coma, and alternatively, hypoglycaemia will also cause permanent CNS damage. There is good evidence that accurate control of blood glucose levels will reduce these complications.

Insulin is produced by the beta cells of the pancreatic islets. It is produced from a precursor molecule (proinsulin); insulin and C-peptide are secreted in equimolar amounts. C-peptide may be a waste product, with no biological activity. In type I diabetes (insulin-dependent), the insulin-secreting cells of the pancreas are destroyed by an immune process, whilst in type II diabetes (non-insulin-dependent), there is diminished insulin secretion and/or end-organ insensitivity. Absolute or relative insulin lack leads to hyperglycaemia and consequent osmotic diuresis, giving rise to thirst, polydipsia, polyuria, electrolyte depletion and weight loss. Intracellular dehydration causes impaired conscious level and increased fat breakdown which leads to ketosis, acidosis and vomiting.

Diabetic Ketoacidosis

This occurs in type I and type II diabetes, either at presentation or with an intercurrent illness, with increased need for insulin. Ketoacidosis is still sometimes fatal. Death is often due to cerebral oedema or hypo/hyperkalaemia. Treatment is aimed at replacing insulin and giving intravenous fluids and potassium. Insulin, preferably by continuous intravenous infusion pump rather than intramuscularly, since absorption may be poor, with peripheral shutdown and acidosis, is started at 6 units/h, falling to 2 units/h when the patient is well enough to eat and drink. A twice-daily s.c. dose (equivalent to that given over the previous 24 h) can then be started. Isotonic saline, with potassium (20 mmol/h), added when plasma K concentrations are known, can be replaced by 5% dextrose or dextrose–saline when the glucose level is below 10 mmol/l. Half-normal saline may be necessary if the plasma sodium is high (above 150 mmol/l), or rises with isotonic saline. There is depletion of body potassium, although initially the plasma K may be high. Bicarbonate is seldom needed, since the acidaemia is corrected by the fluid and insulin replacement. If arterial pH is below 7.0, 50 mmol $NaHCO_3$ may be given i.v., with an additional 10 mmol KCl to counteract the hypokalaemic effect of bicarbonate.

Hyperosmolar Non-ketotic Coma (HONK)

In this disorder of the elderly and West Indians, there is severe hyperglycaemia, sometimes associated with a high sugar-containing drink consumption, a raised urea, high serum osmolarity above 360 mosmol/kg, but no ketosis, probably because of residual insulin secretion. Mortality is high, and there is a high incidence of cerebral venous and arterial thrombosis, and deep vein thrombosis. Treatment is with intravenous insulin as described, but if the patient is hypernatraemic, fluid replacement should be with half-normal saline, and prophylactic heparin adminstration may be necessary. These patients are often very sensitive to small doses of insulin, and in those who survive, hypoglycaemic agents or diet are usually adequate to control symptoms.

In both ketoacidotic coma and HONK, overenthusiastic insulin and fluid replacement can cause cerebral oedema, seen on CT scan, and deterioration in conscious level. Cerebral oedema, poor cerebral blood flow, dehydration and pre-existing vascular occlusion may all account for the high incidence of stroke in these patients.

Hypoglycaemic Coma

The commonest cause of hypoglycaemia is an overdosage of insulin. A low blood glucose leads to signs of high sympathetic activity, with anxiety, palpitations and tremulousness, and sometimes signs of "neuroglycopenia", with odd behaviour, reduced awareness, coma, epilepsy and focal neurological deficits. Diabetics most fear hypoglycaemia when asleep. They may awaken sweating, with headache and poor concentration. If symptoms are not appreciated in time, either glucagon 1 mg i.m. can be given at home by a member of the family, or glucose 20%–50% i.v. can be given in hospital by a doctor. One main danger of prolonged severe hypoglycaemia is cerebral oedema. Mannitol i.v. will improve this rapidly, dexamethasone 4 mg more slowly, but neither drug is very effective, since the main form of oedema here is cytotoxic, with intracellular swelling and not "vasogenic" oedema.

Insulinoma

An insulinoma is a very uncommon cause of hypoglycaemia. Hypoglycaemia in the presence of normal or high insulin levels is diagnostic, since insulin secretion is normally suppressed with hypoglycaemia. These tumours produce very high levels of proinsulin. Cleavage of this molecule is abnormal, and so, although plasma insulin and C-peptide levels are high, they may not be grossly elevated. These assays, if available, are helpful in diagnosis. If spontaneous hypoglycaemia does not occur, a 2-day fast (or fast until hypoglycaemia occurs) may be necessary for diagnosis. Alternatively, exogenous insulin can be given, and the C-peptide response measured. In normal subjects without an insulinoma, C-peptide levels are suppressed.

Angiography and CT scanning find most of these tumours, which are mainly pancreatic. Treatment is by excision, but if this is not possible, if there are metastases, or if the tumour cannot be found, then diazoxide or streptozotocin can be used together with regular meals.

References

Basten A, Pollard JD, Stewart GJ, Frith JA, McLeod JG, Walsh JC, Garrick R, van der Brink CM (1980) Transfer factor in treatment of multiple sclerosis. Lancet II: 931–934

Dowling PC, Bosch VV, Cook SD (1980) Possible beneficial effect of high-dose intravenous steroid therapy in acute demyelinating disease and transverse myelitis. Neurology (Minneap) 30: 33–36

Miller H, Newell DJ, Ridley A (1961) Multiple sclerosis: treatment of acute exacerbations with corticotrophin (ACTH). Lancet II: 1120–1122

Miller JHD, Vas CJ, Naronha MJ, Liversedge LA, Rawson MD (1967) Long-term treatment of multiple sclerosis with corticotrophin. Lancet II: 429–431

Rawson MD, Liversedge LA, Goldfarb G (1966) Treatment of acute retrobular neuritis with corticotrophin. Lancet II: 1044–1046

Rawson MD, Liversedge LA (1969) Treatment of retrobulbar neuritis with corticotrophin. Lancet II: 222

Rosen A, Barsoum AH (1979) Failure of chronic dorsal column stimulation in multiple sclerosis. Ann Neurol 6: 66–67

Saul TG, Ducker TB, Salcman M, Carro E (1981) Steroids in severe head injury: a prospective randomized clinical trial. J Neurosurg 54: 596–600

Suloff MH, Ragatz RE (1982) Hyperbaric oxygenation for the treatment of acute cerebral edema. Neurosurgery 10: 29–38

Tourtelotte WW, Baumhefner RW, Potvin AR, Ma BI, Potrin JH, Mendez M, Syndulko K (1980) Multiple sclerosis de novo CNS IgG synthesis: effect of ACTH and corticosteroids. Neurology (Minneap) 30: 1155–1162

Wiles CW (1982) Steroids in neurology. Br J Hosp Med 28: 308–322

12 Vitamins and the Nervous System

Introduction

With the exception of vitamin B_{12}, folate and thiamine, B-group vitamins and multivitamin preparations are mainly used in neurology as simple, cheap and relatively harmless placebos for patients with an unexplained neuropathy, or with a chronic neurological illness. Despite the lack of evidence of any efficacy here, many vitamins play a vital role in the maintenance of the nervous system. Vitamin A deficiency remains a major cause of blindness in less developed countries, although vitamin A toxicity, due to grossly excessive self-medication, may be commoner than deficiency states in America. In the United Kingdom, pellagra is still seen in lonely old people eating an inadequate diet, and thiamine deficiency, due to alcoholism, is a major health problem throughout the western world. Recently, several reports have suggested that chronic fat malabsorption, resulting in severe and prolonged vitamin E deficiency, can result in spinocerebellar degeneration. Several drugs used in neurology can lead to vitamin deficiency, the best known example being that of pyridoxine deficiency due to isoniazid, although the decarboxylase inhibitors that are widely used in the management of parkinsonism may result in biochemical evidence of niacin depletion, but not clinical pellagra. Vitamin A, vitamin K, niacin and pyridoxine are summarised in Tables 12.1–12.4.

Vitamin B_{12}

The typical patient with addisonian pernicious anaemia has silver-grey hair, with blue eyes and the complexion of an Abernethy biscuit (lemon-yellow: due to haemolytic jaundice). Vitamin B_{12} neuropathy, which may result from any cause of vitamin B_{12} deficiency, is symmetrical, affecting the lower limbs more than upper, and usually presents with paraesthesiae or difficulty in

Table 12.1. Vitamin A

Source	Plant carotenoids
	High content in liver, milk, kidney
Active derivatives	Retinol, retinal, retinoic acid
Function	Formation of visual carotenoid proteins and epithelial glycoproteins
Stores	Total body content 300–900 mg
Deficiency	
Causes	Dietary malnutrition
	Malabsorption
	Liver disease
	Enhanced excretion with proteinuria
Effects	Visual: impaired dark adaptation, abnormal electroretinogram, retinal degeneration, necrosis of cornea (keratomalacia) corneal perforation, blindness
	Epithelial: follicular hyperkeratosis
Treatment	Vitamin A 150 000–300 000 units weekly i.m.
	Prophylaxis 4000 units daily p.o.
Overdosage	
Causes	Arctic explorers with surfeit of polar bear liver
	Carotenaemia
	Food fads
	Theoretical risk of toxicity in breast-fed infants of mothers taking large doses
Effects	Benign raised intracranial pressure
	Hepatomegaly
	High ESR, raised serum calcium and alkaline phosphatase

walking. A neuropathy and also posterior column damage may occur with mild or no anaemia. Neurological features have been attributed to a block in the conversion of homocysteine to methionine with deficiency of S-adenosyl-methionine in the brain. Generalised reversible melanin pigmentation occurs in a few patients with vitamin B_{12} or folate deficiency, but has not been explained.

Main Causes of Vitamin B_{12} Deficiency

1. Intrinsic factor deficiency in addisonian pernicious anaemia is due to a severe autoimmune atrophic gastritis, with failure of intrinsic factor production and circulating anti-parietal cell antibodies in 90% of subjects, anti-intrinsic factor antibodies in 60%. Corticosteroids may reverse gastric atrophy, but do not usually improve vitamin B_{12} absorption.

2. Dietary deficiency is uncommon, with the exception of complete vegans, who may eat no vitamin B_{12}, but usually have a high folate diet. Faulty absorption from the gut is more common than inadequate dietary vitamin B_{12} intake.

3. After total gastrectomy and loss of the intrinsic glycoprotein factor, which is secreted by gastric parietal cells, and is necessary for small bowel

absorption of vitamin B_{12}, depletion of body vitamin B_{12} stores takes 3–5 years. Vitamin B_{12} deficiency may also follow partial gastrectomy, but only after a much longer interval, 10–20 years.

4. Intrinsic factor forms a stable complex with vitamin B_{12} which is absorbed in the lower ileum. Malabsorption, tropical sprue, or virtually any disease of the distal ileum, can cause vitamin B_{12} deficiency.

5. Intense gastric hyperacidity, with a gastrin-secreting tumour (Zollinger–Ellison syndrome) may produce a low intestinal pH and failure of absorption. Vitamin B_{12} malabsorption may also result from the oral hypoglycaemic drug metformin, or neomycin.

6. Large and continuous doses of folic acid may lower the blood concentration of vitamin B_{12}, and in vitamin B_{12} deficiency can precipitate or increase neuropathy, perhaps by reducing the role of vitamin B_{12} in myelin stabilisation, and by increasing vitamin B_{12} utilisation in the catalysis of the formation of tetrahydrofolate from methylfolate. Folic acid, therefore, may cause neurological symptoms of vitamin B_{12} deficiency in subjects who are at risk.

Table 12.2. Vitamin K

Source	Synthesis in the gut (*Escherichia coli*)
Function	γ-Carboxylation of glutamic acid in plasma bone and kidney proteins
	Vitamin K causes resistance to oral anticoagulants (which cause hypoprothrombinaemia by inhibition of the carboxylation of precursor proteins for clotting factors) for 1–2 weeks
Deficiency	
Causes	Newborn and premature infants (lack of gut synthesis from *E. coli*)
	Fat malabsorption
Effects	Failure of formation of clotting factors
Treatment	
1. Oral anticoagulants overdosage with haemorrhage	Phytomenadione 2.5–20 mg slow i.v.
2. Anticoagulant hypoprothrombinaemia, but without haemorrhage	Phytomenadione 10–20 mg p.o.
3. Oral anticoagulant overdosage with haemorrhage, but need to continue anticoagulant (e.g. prosthetic heart valve)	Not vitamin K Fresh frozen plasma, reduce oral anticoagulants
4. Malabsorption	Water-soluble preparation: menadiol sodium diphosphate (avoid in neonates, with risk of kernicterus)

Table 12.3. Niacin

Source	Tryptophan
Active derivatives	Nicotinamide adenine dinucleotide (NAD)
	Nicotinamide adenine dinucleotide phosphate (NADP)
Function	Coenzymes for oxidation and reduction reactions
Deficiency	
Causes	Dietary deficiency
	Disorders of tryptophan metabolism
	Carcinoid syndrome (increased metabolism)
	Hartnup disease (impaired absorption)
	Levodopa with decarboxylase inhibitors (does not cause clinical symptoms)
Effects	Pellagra:
	Hyperkeratotic hyperpigmented skin lesions
	Photosensitivity
	Mental changes, fatigue, insomnia, disorientation, amnesia, psychosis
	Severe diarrhoea
Treatment	Prophylaxis: niacin 10 mg p.o. daily
	Clinical pellagra: niacin 200 mg p.o. 2–3 times daily

Table 12.4. Pyridoxine (vitamin B_6)

Source	Uniformly distributed in all foods
Active derivative	Pyridoxal-5-phosphate
Function	Cofactor for many enzymes involved in amino acid synthesis
	Vital role in neuronal excitability (antiemetic in pregnancy)
Requirements	2 mg daily
	Requirements increased during pregnancy, with oestrogens and with high-protein diet
Deficiency	
Causes	Drugs (inhibit pyridoxal-5-phosphate formation, antagonise its action or increase its excretion) e.g. aminosalicylic acid, pyrazinamide, penicillamine, isoniazid, cycloserine, oestrogens
	Alcoholism
Effects	EEG abnormalities within 3 days
	Generalised seizures, hypsarrhythmia
	Peripheral neuritis, synovial swelling, carpal tunnel syndrome
	Myelitis, encephalitis
	Seborrhoea, stomatitis, glossitis; 30% of alcoholics have biochemical pyridoxine deficiency
Treatment	Prophylaxis in pregnancy, with isoniazid and with oestrogens: pyridoxine 50 mg daily; with penicillamine 150 mg daily
Overdosage	Pyridoxine inhibits central effects of levodopa, perhaps by increasing peripheral decarboxylation to dopamine
	No interaction with Sinemet or Madopar

7. Vitamin B_{12} deficiency has been considered to make patients unduly sensitive to retinal or optic nerve damage by tobacco. However, optic neuritis occasionally occurs in nonsmokers with pernicious anaemia, and hydroxo-

cobalamine given to patients with tobacco amblyopia may restore haematology to normal, but rarely improves vision. The theory that inactivation of cobalamine as cyanocobalamine by smoking or dietary factors results in optic atrophy, or severe neuropathy is no longer tenable.

Chemistry of Vitamin B$_{12}$

Vitamin B$_{12}$ consists of a nucleotide linked to four pyrrol rings with a cobalt atom attached. Attached to the cobalt atom may be cyanide (cyanocobalamine), hydroxyl (hydroxocobalamine), methyl (methylcobalamine) or adenosyl (adenosylcobalamine). The last two are the active forms. Cobalamine in nature is formed by microorganisms, with rich sources in liver, kidney and heart.

Cobalamines are required for nucleic acid synthesis, and vitamin B$_{12}$ is necessary for normal erythropoiesis. Deficiency causes degenerative changes in the spinal cord, central nervous system, peripheral and perhaps optic nerve, with or without megaloblastic anaemia. Only minute daily amounts of vitamin B$_{12}$ (about 1 μg) are required in the diet. The total body stores are about 3 mg.

Plasma Vitamin B$_{12}$ Levels

Vitamin B$_{12}$ is transported by two plasma proteins, transcobalamines I and II. The normal plasma vitamin B$_{12}$ range is 160–900 μg/ml. High values occur in liver disease and myeloproliferative disorders. Over 90% of the vitamin is plasma-bound.

Treatment of Vitamin B$_{12}$ Deficiency

Two forms of vitamin B$_{12}$ are available, cyanocobalamine and hydroxocobalamine. Hydroxocobalamine, although less rapidly absorbed when given i.m., is more effectively stored in the liver. From a 1-mg injection, 15% of cyanocobalamine, but 70% of hydroxocobalamine, is retained. Hydroxocobalamine is now the preparation of choice.

Since hydroxocobalamine has no known toxicity, it is sometimes given in very large doses, 1000 μg vitamin B$_{12}$ daily i.m. for 10 days, and then once weekly in the presence of neurological features of deficiency. However, much lower doses, 500 μg every 2–3 months, are sufficient to replenish body stores in uncomplicated pernicious anaemia, and should be given prophylactically after total gastrectomy, or total ileal resection.

The treatment of megaloblastic anaemia with vitamin B$_{12}$ has been associated with a high incidence of sudden deaths of unknown cause. Hypokalaemia may be a contributory factor, particularly in patients with heart failure on digitalis, in whom plasma potassium levels should be monitored.

Oral or Parenteral Vitamin B$_{12}$ Treatment?

A very small proportion, approximately 1%–2% of an orally administered dose of vitamin B$_{12}$, is absorbed by passive diffusion, and massive daily oral doses of vitamin B$_{12}$ are sometimes effective in the treatment of deficiency, but this is very expensive, unreliable, and needs constant supervision. Resistance to oral doses of vitamin B$_{12}$ may occur in juvenile pernicious anaemia, and oral treatment is therefore indicated only in the very few subjects who develop an allergic response to vitamin B$_{12}$ injection.

Hydroxocobalamine s.c. or i.m. is rapidly and completely absorbed and causes a sense of wellbeing, with reversal of haematological features within days, although neurological improvement is slower. Improvement is independent of the cause of deficiency, whether due to pernicious anaemia, malabsorption due to regional enteritis, Whipple's disease, tuberculosis, intestinal strictures, diverticulosis, anastomosis or tropical sprue (the fish tapeworm *Diphylobothrium latum* as a cause of vitamin B$_{12}$ deficiency has virtually disappeared in Finland).

Folate

The main clinical features of megaloblastic anaemia due to folate deficiency are similar to those when the anaemia is due to vitamin B$_{12}$ deficiency, although the neurological features of the two deficiency states are different. Psychiatric disturbances are more common in folate than in vitamin B$_{12}$ deficiency, whilst a peripheral neuropathy and symptoms of subacute combined degeneration of the spinal cord are less common in folate than in vitamin B$_{12}$ deficiency. The suggestion that folate deficiency may precipitate fits in epilepsy has not been confirmed.

Folic Acid

Folic acid occurs in all green plants, and is also present in a wide variety of animal tissues. It is the precursor of the coenzyme tetrahydrofolic acid, concerned with the transfer of single carbon units, and in the formation of DNA, and is made up of a glutamic acid–pteridine conjugate linked via *p*-aminobenzoic acid.

Between 30% and 50% of total body folate is stored in the liver, and 60% of plasma folate is protein-bound. The red cell folate content gives a more accurate index of body stores than plasma folate levels, which fluctuate with dietary intake. Folate is concentrated in the cerebrospinal fluid, where levels are 3–4 times higher than in plasma. Body folate stores last 2–4 months, and folate deficiency therefore develops more rapidly than vitamin B$_{12}$ deficiency.

Causes of Folate Deficiency

1. Anticonvulsant drugs cause folate deficiency. These impair folate absorption, increase folate utilisation by hepatic microsomal enzymes, and inhibit the hydrolytic enzymes which release the folic acid from conjugates in vegetables. High folate doses do not cause convulsions in normal people. If clinical symptoms of folate deficiency occur in people with epilepsy on anticonvulsants, folate supplements should be given. However, folic acid therapy may cause a fall in plasma phenytoin level.

2. Although antiepileptic drugs are the main cause of folate deficiency in neurological practice, other drugs such as the antineoplastic drug methotrexate and the antimalarial drug pyrimethamine also cause folate deficiency. In these instances, deficiency should be treated with folinic rather than folic acid to bypass the block that prevents folate utilisation.

3. Folate deficiency may be nutritional in old people living on tea and toast, and also in alcoholics, or be due to malabsorption in tropical sprue, coeliac syndromes or diseases of the small intestine. A number of rare hereditary disorders of the specific absorption mechanism for folate are known, and may cause ataxia, mental handicap and megaloblastic anaemia.

4. Symptoms of folate deficiency sometimes result from excessive utilisation in pregnancy, with an inadequate diet, and also occur in malignant disease.

Symptoms of Folate Deficiency

Folate deficiency causes neuropathy and altered behaviour, as well as megaloblastic anaemia. There are unequivocal reports of myelopathy in subjects with low folate, but normal plasma vitamin B_{12} levels.

Treatment of Folate Deficiency

Folate deficiency is treated by replacement with oral folic acid 1–5 mg daily. Orally administered folate is absorbed throughout the gut, mainly in the small intestine. Doses as high as 15 mg are fully absorbed.

Treatment causes a reticulocyte response in 4–5 days, but improvement in neuropathy when due to folate deficiency is much slower. Folic acid will also improve the haematological, but not the neurological features of vitamin B_{12} deficiency. Prophylaxis with folic acid should be given in chronic malnutrition and in alcoholism, as well as in pregnancy. Folic acid has no effect in people who are not folate-deficient.

Thiamine

The major causes of thiamine deficiency include malnutrition and alcoholism. The clinical presentation of thiamine deficiency is determined by the presence of malnutrition, and by lack of other vitamins. Largely dependent on these factors, thiamine deficiency is associated with beriberi, alcoholic and pregnancy neuritis, Wernicke's encephalopathy or Korsakoff's psychosis. Acute deficiency in any of these conditions should be treated with thiamine hydrochloride 250 mg i.v.

The response to thiamine in infantile beriberi is one of the most rapid and dramatic in medicine; and the ophthalmoplegia of Wernicke's disease may also improve within a few hours of thiamine administration, although other lesions of the brain and spinal cord related to thiamine deficiency are slow to recover with treatment.

A few rare inborn errors of metabolism result in chronic thiamine deficiency. Here, thiamine replacement may improve megaloblastic anaemia, lactic acidosis, branched-chain ketoaciduria, and intermittent cerebellar ataxia.

Leigh's disease (subacute necrotising encephalomyelopathy), although mainly occurring in infants, has an extremely diverse presentation, and also occurs in adults. The concentration of thiamine triphosphate in neuronal tissue is low, and thiamine phosphorylation is inhibited. In some cases, massive doses of thiamine hydrochloride have reportedly caused a dramatic improvement in neurological status, but the effect is not sustained, and the usual clinical response of patients with Leigh's disease to pharmacological doses of thiamine is minor.

Thiamine occurs in nerve axons. Thiamine is a coenzyme in the oxidative decarboxylation of α-ketoacids, ketoglutarate and pyruvate, and has a specific role in nerve conduction. All plant and animal cells require thiamine as a coenzyme for decarboxylase. Thiamine is present in many plant and animal foods, in high concentration in the outer coat of grains, but is lost in the preparation of white flour or polished rice.

Thiamine is necessary for the maintenance of the peripheral and central nervous system. The pentose phosphate pathway is thiamine-dependent, and is necessary for lipid synthesis. Thiamine deficiency may lead to peripheral demyelination by blockade of this pathway.

The absorption and metabolism of thiamine is influenced by the carbohydrate intake. Therefore, intravenous glucose should not be given without thiamine to alcoholics, since this may precipitate deficiency syndromes. Intestinal absorption is limited to 8–15 mg thiamine per day. This is achieved by taking 40 mg in divided oral doses. The normal daily thiamine requirement is less than this, approximately 1 mg, a similar amount being excreted as pyrimidine in the urine.

There is an increased requirement for thiamine in pregnancy, and some foods, e.g. fresh fish, clams and mussels, contain thiaminases which destroy the vitamin.

Vitamin E

Vitamin E, α-tocopherol, has long been an orphan amongst vitamins, with no clear function in humans. In animals with experimentally induced vitamin E deficiency, posterior column degeneration and peripheral neuropathy occur. Similar changes sometimes occur in human malabsorption syndromes, mainly in children. In these conditions, dysarthria, ophthalmoplegia, pigmentary retinal changes, generalised muscle weakness, extensor plantar responses and superficial sensory loss occur. A dying-back neuropathy in sensory neurones, and degenerative changes in the spinocerebellar tracts, occur, and have been attributed to lack of vitamin E, although there may be little or no clinical response to vitamin E supplementation. Very rarely, vitamin E deficiency also occurs in patients who do not have generalised fat malabsorption, but perhaps a specific failure of vitamin E absorption (Harding et al. 1985).

Low serum vitamin E concentrations have been documented in children with cystic fibrosis, coeliac disease, biliary atresia, abetalipoproteinaemia, intestinal lymphangiectasia and following extensive intestinal resection. Oral treatment with vitamin E given in massive amounts (270 mg kg^{-1} day^{-1}), or using an oral water-miscible preparation (α-tocopherol polyethyleneglycol succinate, 75–900 units/day) may result in an increase in serum vitamin E levels. In cystic fibrosis, serum vitamin E levels may return to normal values.

Abetalipoproteinaemia represents the most severe form of vitamin E deficiency known. Massive doses of vitamin E (100 mg kg^{-1} day^{-1}) are needed here to maintain normal serum concentrations, but there is no improvement in the progressive disabling spinocerebellar and peripheral nerve disorder, despite oral vitamin E therapy. In other forms of vitamin E deficiency, long-term prospective studies are needed to see if vitamin E will prevent the appearance of posterior column and peripheral nerve lesions. Once present, posterior column damage may be largely irreversible.

In a child with long-standing vitamin E deficiency associated with malabsorption due to cholestatic liver disease, reported by Rosenblum et al. (1981) liver transplant did not improve either the severe neurological handicap or serum vitamin E levels.

In summary, there is increasing evidence that vitamin E deficiency, usually due to generalised fat malabsorption, can result in a progressive neurological syndrome of ataxia, areflexia and loss of proprioception. However, vitamin E therapy may not be curative, at least in the established illness. Serum vitamin E concentrations should be determined early in spinocerebellar syndromes, particularly those that develop in childhood or early adult life, and despite the present lack of clear evidence of efficacy, replacement vitamin E treatment should be given.

References

Harding AE, Matthews S, Jones S, Ellis CJK, Booth SW, Muller DRR (1985) Spinocerebellar degeneration associated with a selective defect of vitamin E absorption. New Engl J Med 313: 32–35

Rosenblum JL, Keating JP, Prensky AL, Nelson JS (1981) A progressive neurologic syndrome in children with chronic liver disease. New Engl J Med 304: 503–508

Subject Index